A WOMAN'S
WALK WITH GOD

To order additional copies of *A Woman's Walk With God,* by Ginger Mostert Church, call 1-800-765-6955.

Visit us at www.reviewandherald.com for information on other Review and Herald® products.

Ginger Church

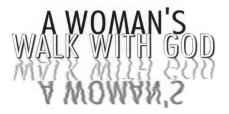

A WOMAN'S WALK WITH GOD

Finding Balance for Body and Soul

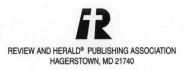

REVIEW AND HERALD® PUBLISHING ASSOCIATION
HAGERSTOWN, MD 21740

This book was
Edited by Jocelyn Fay
Copyedited by Jocelyn Fay and James Cavil
Designed by Freshcut Design
Cover photo by Jerome Tisne/Getty Images
Electronic makeup by Shirley M. Bolivar
Typeset: 11/14 Stempel Schneidler

PRINTED IN U.S.A.

08 07 06 05 04   5 4 3 2 1

R&H Cataloging Service
Church, Ginger Mostert
    A woman's walk with God: finding balance for body and soul.

    1. Women—Religious life. I. Title.

                248.843

ISBN 0-8280-1795-6

FOR YOU,
DENNIS, DOUG, AND DONY

I have found myself in the midst of so many adventures, climbing higher than I felt comfortable, speaking when I would have felt much better keeping quiet, simply because the three of you are, and have always been, encouragers. Whether singly or together, you have pressed me to go beyond what I felt comfortable doing to what you felt God wanted me to do.

Your faith in me, when I procrastinated instead of starting to write this book, made all the difference between an idea that would have slowly faded away and a manuscript written expressly to bless others.

Your willingness to set up our computer and a cozy office so I would have no excuses should have been inspiration enough. Yet it took numerous gentle nudges from the three of you and your continued inquiries as to whether I'd started yet and how far I'd actually gotten to finally push me into writing this book.

A wife and mother couldn't have been more blessed, and I thank God continually for each of you.

YOU
WEREN'T ALONE

What an opportunity came into my life 22 years ago, when I went to work for the Review and Herald Publishing Association—spending time with giants in the field of writing and editing, such as Kenneth Wood, William Johnsson, and Robert Spangler. Being encouraged to write and receiving instruction and encouragement from Aileen Andres Sox, Jocelyn Fay, Penny Estes Wheeler, and Marie Spangler. These people have made a world of difference for me.

Writing? In those days it never entered my mind! I soon found, though, that those who can write are eager to share their love of the written word and to encourage others to try their hand at crafting material that can and will change lives! These caring editors and writers have built and molded people everywhere for service with a dedication and intenseness that I find impossible to describe.

Later I would also be privileged to work with Chris Blake, Dan Fahrbach, Kim and Lori Peckham, Kris Coffin Stevenson, Stuart Tyner, Harold and Rose Otis, and Larry Becker. Each of you have touched my life in a unique way and encouraged me to "learn more," "try," "try harder," and then "try again."

Finally, I thank Jeannette Johnson and her team for "being there." Her encouragement, trust, and e-mails resulted in this finished manuscript.

To each of you I say, "Thank you." I now work tirelessly to pass on to others everything that you have taught me. Over the years many other people have given of their time, energy, and knowledge to help me discover the joys of writing—to each of you, whose names are too numerous to mention, I also say, "Thank you."

CONTENTS

BEVERLY, IF YOU HAD ONLY KNOWN
THE AGONY YOU WOULD CAUSE ME . . .

God led Beverly Holweger to push my faith to the limit. That day, in the early months of 2002, she called to invite me to do a seminar at her women's retreat. I said, "Yes!" She responded with the heart-stopping words, "Our committee has chosen the subject 'A Woman and Her Devotions' for you to present."

I instantly had second thoughts.

"You've chosen the wrong person," I hurriedly responded.

But Beverly wouldn't take no for an answer.

I prayed. I agonized. I lost sleep. I pleaded with God to talk to me—to show me what to say. Two months passed.

The appointed weekend came closer. Nothing fell into place.

Just before despair overtook me, God spoke to me. I awoke that morning and headed to the shower as usual. Just as I closed the door, inspiration hit. *Talk about the eight laws of health!* The voice in my head spoke so clearly that I hurried to my nightstand and reached for my trusty pen and pad of paper. I began to write furiously. Fifteen minutes later the outline lay before me.

But as I reread the written words and realized what they said, I again cried out to God: "I can't share this! They will know, all of them will see, that I don't practice what I preach. What can I do? You must have made a mistake! I struggle so with my devotional life. How can I face them?"

I gave that seminar. Yet I tell you honestly that when I returned home, Dennis and I began to make changes. Serious, life-changing things that were not easy. We have never looked back. God is good! I share with you not from anything I have done, but from knowledge of what God will do for you.

INTRODUCTION

Where Are You Going, Enoch?

*"After he begot Methuselah, Enoch walked with God three hundred years,
and had sons and daughters. So all the days of Enoch were three hundred and
sixty-five years. And Enoch walked with God; and he was not, for God took him"*
(Genesis 5:22-24).

Imagine setting out on a journey with no destination in
mind. In fact, you feel so strongly about choosing your own
way that you fail even to bring along the necessary supplies
to make your trip enjoyable. Because you have no particular plan in mind, the clothes in your suitcase soon prove to
be inadequate. At each junction you wish you had a map,
but you don't purchase one for fear that just taking a peek
will put someone else in control.

A nightmare? Not a situation you want to find yourself
in? Each of us arrives at a journey—a life to be lived. The
Bible gives the length of time we are given as 70 years. "And
if by reason of strength they are eighty years, yet their boast
is only labor and sorrow" (Psalm 90:10). None of us chooses
where or how our lives will begin, although God knows
(Jeremiah 1:5). We came into this world sinful (Romans
3:23) and helpless. So what are you doing with the life
you've been given? Do you long to enter into the Enoch experience—a life of walking and talking with God? What
would it be like to have God as our constant companion?
Can you imagine walking with Him closer and closer
toward your heavenly home?

Perhaps your life feels hopeless. You have experienced

untold suffering at the hands of another. Abuse and neglect came to you from those very individuals who should have given you only love and care. Could your life, even now, be a nightmare of pain, sickness, or sorrow as you struggle to live faithfully each day?

Perhaps you've been given every advantage. It could be that you have enjoyed loving parents, a Christian education, and close friendships. Yet no matter how hard you try, deep inside you feel that nothing you ever have done or ever will do can measure up to the goals of perfection and service that are ever before you. What then? Should you just throw up your hands and declare that all is hopeless?

Let's take a trip back to the beginning of the world. God created a garden. The Bible tells us that "God made every tree grow that is pleasant to the sight and good for food" (Genesis 2:9). What a home! Perfect in every way, and beautiful to behold. What could go wrong there? If only you and I had been placed in this setting. Wait . . . What's happening? Eve has walked over to the forbidden tree, the tree of knowledge of good and evil. She's talking to an exquisite serpent there! Just last evening she and Adam spent quality time with God. They walked and talked in the garden with Him, finishing yet another day of pleasant work and the excellent company of God's created beings. What is Eve doing? I must turn my head away. *Don't touch the fruit, Eve! Leave it alone! Run . . . run . . . Eve, you will ruin everything!*

You know the story. Eve listened when she should have walked away. She caved in! She reached out her hand and took the fruit that the serpent promised would keep her from dying, would open her eyes and make her like God (Genesis 3:4, 5). You and I are not privileged to know why Eve hurried to Adam and offered him the forbidden morsel. Did she realize the horror of her mistake and seek Adam's approval and assurance that she had not messed up her life? Could she feel a sense of power that she wanted to share with him?

We can only surmise the events that took place over the next moments, hours, and days. We do know from the Bible story that in the cool of the day God called Adam and Eve—and found them hiding (verses 8-10). Thus began the sinful journey of men and women everywhere. Food tripped up our earthly parents: a wrong choice made and a forbidden bite taken and shared. Misery untold resulted for all men, women, and children who would follow.

Through the pages of this book we will study the Christian's walk with God and how it relates not only to our choice of what we will eat, but to all of the eight laws of health.* Does one have bearing on the other? Can we triumph in our daily life and ignore these powerful suggestions for success?

Obey one and see a difference. Embrace two or three and experience new power and zest. Make all a part of your daily living and find yourself walking the walk of Enoch— "And Enoch walked with God; and he was not, for God took him" (Genesis 5:24).

---

*Ellen White lists them this way: "Pure air, sunlight, abstemiousness, rest, exercise, proper diet, the use of water, trust in divine power" (*The Ministry of Healing,* p. 127).

Chapter One

GET OUT OF THE BOX

Let the Cleanliness and Fragrance of Fresh Air Into Your Life.

～

*Close your eyes and get comfortable. Well, as comfortable as you
can in your present surroundings. Try to ignore the smallness of the room you
inhabit and its lack of ventilation. You will soon discover a disconcerting fact:
This room is not heated in the winter or air-conditioned in the summer.
The windows do not open, and the door is closed with a seal to keep
out any draft. How does it feel? How long can you and I maintain a
healthy lifestyle without the first of our eight laws of health—fresh air?*

As soon as you can claw, scratch, or beg your way out
of the sealed room, it's human nature for you to take a
deep breath. In fact, many cleansing, life-giving breaths.
No longer do you take air, that amazing substance you
previously took for granted, into your lungs without giving it thought. *What would happen to me if I couldn't get air?*
you ponder.

In our Christian experience we also need the cleanliness
and fragrance of life-giving "air." We are buried under layers
of sin, disillusionment, and regret. But peel away those layers and free ourselves of the stench of sin, and suddenly the
fragrance of God's love wafts into us and all around us.

What steps do you need to take to assure yourself of an
unlimited supply of fresh air?

Face your fears and faults.

Our human nature often makes us react to anything out
of the ordinary by turning and running. Perhaps if we can
get far enough away from our fear, it will disappear. The

Bible paints a different picture. We find in 1 John 1:9: "If we confess our sins, He is faithful and just to forgive us our sins and to cleanse us from all unrighteousness." Again we find, "He who covers his sins will not prosper, but whoever confesses and forsakes them will have mercy" (Proverbs 28:13). And again, "Confess your trespasses to one another, and pray for one another, that you may be healed" (James 5:16).

When we face our fears, often we uncover the faults that we have so carefully hidden and harbored. Suddenly, taken out into the light, theses faults almost overwhelm us. But God asks us to work out our own salvation, "that you may become blameless and harmless, children of God without fault in the midst of a crooked and perverse generation, among whom you shine as lights in the world" (Philippians 2:15).

Now, as we've faced our faults and confessed our sins, we find an assurance that liberates us from fear. "For God has not given us a spirit of fear, but of power and of love and of a sound mind" (2 Timothy 1:7).

Find time alone with God.

From the beginning, God has made time to be with His children. "In the cool of the day" God walked with Adam and Eve (Genesis 3:8). Face-to-face, through dreams, through messengers, through His word—in all these ways God has communicated with those He created and loves.

The hymn says, "Take time to be holy, speak oft with thy Lord." How do you guard your time so that you can speak often with God? Some treasure the hours between 4:00 and 5:00 a.m. as the best times of fellowship with Him. Others, like me, are not at their best during these hours and struggle to find another way to commune with Him.

You may enjoy prayer walks—giving family, friends, leaders, and others you care about to God with singing, prayer, and praise. Take advantage of times when you are sitting at a traffic light, stopped behind a school bus, or in a slow line at the supermarket. (For more tips on making your time with God more special, see Appendix A.)

It takes only a desire and an action to commune with God. As you study to show yourself approved (2 Timothy 2:15), you will enjoy harmony with Christ. Fellowship with God will bring you continuing joy, because you will find that you and He are of one accord.

Freely speak to God when you communicate with Him.

Have you ever tried to carry on a conversation with someone while at the same time trying to hide information from them that might put you in a bad light? Probably you both felt awkward. Yet how often do you try to hide things from God? Perhaps you feel a need to cover your feelings of anger, despair, unworthiness, and loneliness. Do you hesitate to talk of disillusionment and grief with your Creator and Friend?

The Bible tells stories of men and women who, when speaking with Jesus, honestly voiced their concerns and sorrows. Job, through his ordeal of suffering and loss, kept his mind and heart turned to his Savior. In the midst of his pain he proclaimed to his friends, "Even today my complaint is bitter; my hand is listless because of my groaning. Oh, that I knew where I might find Him" (Job 23:2, 3).

David cried out to God, "Why do You stand afar off, O Lord? Why do You hide in times of trouble?" (Psalm 10:1). In his times of chastening he pleaded, "O Lord, do not rebuke me in Your wrath, nor chasten me in Your hot displeasure!" (Psalm 38:1). In times of distress he proclaimed, "As the deer pants for the water brooks, so pants my soul for You, O God" (Psalm 42:1). David spoke to God honestly and from his heart. How can we do less?

Have you ever wanted something so bad that you could "taste it?" Perhaps you wanted a different job more suited to your skills. Even as it slipped from your grasp you pleaded with the Lord, "I deserve better." Maybe your heart's desire is a close friend, a life partner, or renewed health. Talk honestly to God with assurance that He hears and answers all of our prayers—often in ways you and I don't understand.

Dennis and I had just moved to Nashville, Tennessee. *How exciting,* I thought. *What a blessing if we could only buy a beautiful new house.* Deep in my heart I knew we deserved one—hadn't we followed God's call in this move, and wouldn't He want our family to finally have a great new place?

Then we found my idea of the perfect place to raise our boys. I'd already talked to God about our needs and desires, and then we just happened upon it. *Now, if only I could get Dennis excited about it. If only he would agree and see buying it God's and my way.*

"Ginger," Dennis said, hesitating because he knew my level of anticipation, "I'll have a very long commute on a busy highway from here. Are you sure this house is right for us?"

"Help me persuade him, Jesus," I whispered. "Don't let him be difficult and make us miss this perfect part of Your plan for us."

"I'm afraid it's awfully small," Dennis continued. "We wouldn't even have a basement. And what about storage?"

Armed with the knowledge that God would not want to withhold any good thing from us, I finally brought Dennis around to see the good things about the house. We signed on the dotted line.

Among the host of words in that contract was one sentence that gave us a grace period of three days to come up with the funds if the seller found another buyer, and we had not sold our other house.

Paper signed, contract in hand, we drove quietly back across town. Each of us was lost in our own private thoughts.

"I hope we're doing the right thing," Dennis worried aloud. "I don't really feel good about this . . ."

Had I boldly put my wants into Gods plan? Why didn't I listen to my husband and his doubts? Again I pleaded with God, "Now what will we do? If only . . ."

We walked through the door of our rented place to a ringing telephone. From Dennis's half of the conversation I knew he was talking to our real estate agent, and the news wasn't good. "You say he won't accept our contract? . . . You'll have to give us our deposit back? . . . You don't know why he's acting this way? . . . It's never happened to you before?"

Often we don't understand. The home God ultimately led us to fit our needs so much better. A loving God had heard my prayer. He had not punished my exuberance and strong will, but led us in a better way. The patience of God and His desire for our good taught me an enduring lesson that day.

Whether you are experiencing times of joy and renewal or enduring days of pain and peril, you can talk to God as to a friend. Believe what the Bible says when you read that nothing can separate us from the love of Christ (Romans 8:35-39). It's a promise you can bank on.

Face the future.

Have you ever tried to walk forward while looking backward? It doesn't work. Imagine flying down the highway, moving in and out of traffic, with your eyes fixed on the rearview mirror. Truthfully, your trip would be a very short one, ending in dented fenders and flared tempers. It's important to watch where you're going! In fact, you can't do otherwise and survive.

The same principle applies to our life today. You must remember what God has done on your behalf and remind yourself of your blessings. Yet you cannot continue forward without looking in that direction. Just as the Israelites went forward through the Red Sea even though it seemed impossible, you must face the future unafraid, knowing that God will not leave you alone (Hebrews 13:5).

How often do you let your mind wander to times of disappointment and missed opportunities? When "if only" and "I wonder" cause you to falter, let them go! These roadblocks to joyful living are Satan's ploy to turn your heart from God.

Feel **exalted and free.**

No longer do you go to bed at night or arise in the morning bearing the heavy burden of guilt. Suddenly you are free. No need to hold on to memories of regret and shame. You have placed them at Jesus' feet. You have a great future in Christ. Each new day will find you eager and ready to make a difference. Satan no longer has you bound in despair. He can tempt you. He *will* tempt you! Yet, you walk, talk, and enjoy fellowship with the God of the universe. You go forward dwelling in the secret place of God's tabernacle (Psalm 27:5).

Find **faith and joy.**

It's a promise. "The apostles said to the Lord, 'Increase our faith.' So the Lord said, 'If you have faith as a mustard seed, you can say to this mulberry tree, "Be pulled up by the roots and be planted in the sea," and it would obey you'" (Luke 17:5, 6). Faith abounds in the Bible. Children have it.

Young men and old reach out with assurance. Women hold on to faith as heaven and earth seem to fail them.

Faith heals those who are blind and leprous. Faith causes a lame man to walk. "Faith comes by hearing" (Romans 10:17). Paul says, "I have fought the good fight, I have finished the race, I have kept the faith" (2 Timothy 4:7).

And joy . . . "joy comes in the morning" (Psalm 30:5), after the darkness, when the trials and tribulations—the temptations—are overcome and the sick made well. Even when those we love are laid to rest and we need the touch of One who understands, "joy comes in the morning." Suddenly we can "sing for joy" (Isaiah 65:14). The picture has changed. Indecision and hiding are replaced with "joy inexpressible" (1 Peter 1:8). Dirty rags hanging on our bodies suddenly appear to be robes of righteousness.

Are we finished? No, there's still more we can do to enjoy the fresh air of God's love and forgiveness.

Fess up and be cleansed.

"Do not be deceived, God is not mocked; for whatever a man sows, that he will also reap" (Galatians 6:7). But that cannot be the end of the story. First John 1:9 adds to it, "If we confess our sins, He is faithful and just to forgive us our sins and to cleanse us from all unrighteousness."

Not "some of our sins." Not even "a few of our sins." The Bible says "*all* unrighteousness." Confess your sins and let them go. Picture each one sinking to the depths of the sea. Oh, yes, sometimes the results of our sins harm others even to the third and fourth generation. Yet the apostle John says, "My little children, these things I write to you, so that you may not sin. And if anyone sins, we have an Advocate with the Father, Jesus Christ the righteous" (1 John 2:1). Place yourself in that lovely verse that gives so much assurance and hope, "For God so loved the world that He gave His only begotten Son, that whoever [your name] believes in Him should not perish but have everlasting life" (John 3:16).

Don't let the sun go down on your anger or on a wrong you have done. Take time to review your actions at the end of each day. Make amends when you have hurt another. Turn to God with anything that will mar your happiness or steal away your joy. "The steps of a good man are ordered by the Lord, and He delights in his way. Though he fall, he shall not be utterly cast down; for the Lord upholds him with His hand" (Psalm 37:23, 24).

Funnel God's warmth into your life.

Have your ever watched a cat? I love to watch ours, Teddy and Bear, follow a beam of sunlight from one room to the next—from window to floor and floor to couch or chair. God has placed in them the nature to want to feel the warmth and healing power of the sun.

What about you? Are you looking for ways to feel God's warmth? Jesus' secret of success was that he went "to the garden alone." No disruption. Beauty and peace everywhere. "Seek the Lord while He may be found" (Isaiah 55:6).

A life apart from Christ soon turns cold and discouraging. Gone are the promises and encouragement of protection and forgiveness. In their place come accusations and error. Breathe deeply of the fresh air of cleanliness of heart. "Let me have joy from you in the Lord; refresh my heart in the Lord" (Philemon 20). Even as we breathe life-giving air, we realize that we want more. We need more of God's incredible gifts of life. So we hurry on!

Chapter Two

RENEW YOUR LIFE FORCE

Bask in the Glow of Sunshine, the Gift That's Impossible to Hide.

"Awesome" and "amazing" describe the experience of one who lives his or her life in the presence of Christ. Gone is the darkness that surrounds the earth from the evils of sin. In its place you find life in abundance. This second gift, sunshine, comes from a loving Father to those who seek Him and find Him.

Moses had to veil his face when he came into the presence of God. The face of Jesus "shone like the sun" (Matthew 17:2) on the Mount of Transfiguration. Listen to the words of Moses as he blessed the priests: "The Lord bless you and keep you; the Lord make His face shine upon you, and be gracious to You" (Numbers 6:24, 25). And when the apostle John saw the heavenly city, he said that there was "no need of the sun or of the moon to shine in it, for the glory of God illuminated it. The Lamb is its light" (Revelation 21:23).

Can everyone have this special glow? Listen to the words of Matthew: "Let your light so shine before men, that they may see your good works and glorify your Father in heaven" (Matthew 5:16).What a privilege to glorify our Father as we go about our daily lives. It's not only possible for us to have this special gift; it's a promise we've been given: "The glory which You gave Me I have given them, that they may be one just as We are one. . . . Father, I desire that they also whom You gave Me may be with Me where I am, that they may behold My glory which You have given Me; for You loved Me before the foundation of the world" (John 17:22-24).

As humans, many of us are drawn to the light. From sunshine we get vitamin D—a necessary ingredient of health and healing. How dark and dreary are the days of clouds and shadows. Often suicidal thoughts and sickness afflict those who fail to receive enough of the sun's life-giving properties. That's why a Christian must take sunshine seriously and receive all the benefits it brings, both physically and spiritually.

What exactly does it take for the Christian to be illuminated with God's glory on this earth? Here are a few suggestions.

Speak clearly and often with God.

A young woman accepted a much-longed-for position at a local business. The first morning she dressed carefully and arrived at her new office early. Closing her office door, she worked long and hard calling friends with the news of her good fortune. Day after day she labored, focusing on small, insignificant tasks that she felt comfortable with and needed no help in completing. At the end of the first week a gentle knock at the door brought the message that she was wanted in the president's office.

"I've waited for your appearance this week," the president gently admonished. "I had so many plans for you. When you didn't show up, I wondered if you took your talents elsewhere."

"Oh, no!" came the reply. "Had you looked into my office, you would have seen just how busy I was."

"How so?" pressed the surprised administrator. "The list of tasks our firm needs you to accomplish lies untouched in your basket on my desk."

Our young friend is not alone. It's easy to find ourselves so busy that we neglect the most important thing—meeting with God. Do you find time daily, hourly, moment by moment to speak with Him? Is it your practice to listen for that still small voice that often instructs you in the way that you should go?

The boy Samuel thought he was hearing the voice of Eli; in time he found it to be the voice of God.

Consider Hagar as she wept for herself and her son in the midst of their suffering, shame, and despair. "The angel of God called to Hagar out of heaven, and said to her, 'What ails you, Hagar? Fear not, for God has heard the voice of the lad where he is'" (Genesis 21:17).

Noah, Abraham, Moses, Joshua, Jonah, Job, Stephen, Saul, Peter, Mary, and Martha . . . the list of Bible personalities is endless. Those who followed Jesus communicated with Him. Each shared what was in their heart and listened for His response. No matter what the circumstances—in good times or evil—these biblical people show us how to walk and talk with God. We learn from them that listening is as important as speaking, for walking ahead of God's leading brings only disaster, and following too far behind leads to missed opportunities.

Jesus told his followers a hard saying, "As the living Father sent Me, and I live because of the Father, so he who feeds on Me will live because of Me" (John 6:57). Many turned away, not understanding how Jesus could be "life." Verse 63 says, "It is the Spirit who gives life. . . . The words that I speak to you are spirit, and they are life."

Share **His warmth with others.**

It's an amazing and wonderful thing to be filled with the warmth of God's love. Basking in God's presence fills you with so much warmth that it must be shared. You cannot continue as if nothing has happened. "You shall receive power when the Holy Spirit has come upon you; and you shall be witnesses to Me in Jerusalem, and in all Judea and Samaria, and to the end of the earth" (Acts 1:8).

After Jesus healed the blind men He warned, "'See that no one knows it.' But when they had departed, they spread the news about Him in all that country" (Matthew 9:30, 31).

Is it possible that God's warmth, His healing touch, can reach and change you without your telling others? No. Good news must be shared!

Show **your gratitude in words and actions.**

Genuine appreciation—a realization that your life will never be the same—brings renewed vigor and focus. What if God had not reached out to you? Where would you be without His love and forgiveness? Questions such as these cause you to shudder as you visualize life without this Redeemer and Friend.

Saul, after Christ confronted him on the road to Damascus, became transformed into the zealous apostle Paul, who devoted the remainder of his life to serving others. "I have been crucified with Christ," he said. "It is no longer I who live, but Christ lives in me; and the life which I now live in the flesh I live by faith in the Son of God, who loved me and gave Himself for me" (Galatians 2:20).

Dorcas worked tirelessly for others. The good Samaritan accepted no payment for saving a robbery victim's life. Anyone who knows Jesus, who experiences His touch, wants to pass it on—to bless others.

Shower **Him with your love.**

"What does God want from us first and foremost? Well, what does a parent want from a child, or a pet owner from a pet? Perfection? Service? No. Love. What God wants from us, first and foremost, is our companionship, our affection. Sometimes God must feel like the proverbial lonely wife whose husband is always off making money but never has time for his bride. God wants us to spend time with Him before we work hard for Him. *He wants us to purr in His lap"* (Tim Crosby, Ruthie Jacobsen, and Lonnie Melashenko, *A Passion for Prayer,* p. 8).

"The first words of Scripture are 'In the beginning God.' That is a recipe for spiritual success" (*ibid.,* p. 9). The widow gave her mite. She gave God her all. Mary washed Jesus' feet with fine perfume and dried them with her hair. She gave Him her best. Can you and I do less?

Men and women of the Bible glorified God and spilled out their love in an unending variety of ways. Each trusted God as their friend. Fear was not an ingredient of their relationship. Love and trust drew them to the Eternal One.

"Then Moses and the children of Israel sang this song to the Lord, and spoke, saying: 'I will sing to the Lord, for He has triumphed gloriously! The horse and its rider He has thrown into the sea! The Lord is my strength and song, and He has become my salvation; He is my God, and I will praise Him; my father's God, and I will exalt Him. The Lord is a man of war; the Lord is His name'" (Exodus 15:1-3).

Speak **of Him to others.**

What if you were to come home from a hard day's work to find that your husband had arrived home two hours earlier? You might not think anything about it except for one thing: Before you arrived he had worked like a whirlwind. He not only cleaned the kitchen (including mopping the floor) but also vacuumed the entire house. Now, as you walk through the door, you are met with the exciting aroma of your favorite dinner.

Is it even remotely possible that you wouldn't tell anyone about your good fortune? Only two questions remain: How many people will you tell about your wonderful surprise? and How soon you will start telling them? And wouldn't you also spread the word if you found shoes at half price or a furniture store going out of business? Men and women alike enjoy sharing stories of good fortune. Watch a child who has something new—they often tremble from the joy and excitement.

Now consider that Christian who says, "I just can't share anything about Jesus. You know, I'm shy. Sharing Jesus isn't my talent." Should you find yourself speaking these words or others like them, let me give you a few questions to mull over:

1. Am I in love with Jesus, or do I know very little about Him?
2. Which word do I use the most often when something good happens to me, "blessed" or "lucky"?
3. When was the last time I got excited enough about anything to share it with others?
4. Am I still breathing—or just living dead?
5. If today were my last day on earth, would that make it any easier for me to share with others what God has done in my life?
6. How often do I thank God for His blessings?
7. How many blessings have I been given this week? (Perhaps you should begin a list and create something to be excited about.)
8. Am I ungrateful for other blessings besides spiritual ones?
9. How bad would it be if I told someone about God and they didn't listen, or worse yet, mocked me?

Ask yourself, *How many chapters or verses can I read in the*

Gospels before coming across an excited person? "I've found a pearl!" "My son has returned home—let's have a feast!" "I'm healed—I can run, walk, jump, speak, live!" "I'm alive!" Do you understand? If you and I find sharing so hard, most likely it goes back to our weak Christian experience. We just don't feel we have anything of importance to talk about.

Paul, writing to the Corinthians, tells of having a disability of some kind. Three times he asked God to remove it. Each time God's answer was "My grace is enough; it's all you need. My strength comes into its own in your weakness" (2 Corinthians 12:8, 9, Message). Paul continues, "Once I heard that, I was glad to let it happen. I quit focusing on the handicap and began appreciating the gift [the disability]. It was a case of Christ's strength moving in on my weakness. Now I take limitations in stride, and with good cheer, these limitations that cut me down to size—abuse, accidents, opposition, bad breaks. I just let Christ take over! And so the weaker I get, the stronger I become" (verses 9, 10, Message).

When you *must* share what God has done for you—the love you feel for Him—you will know that you are walking with God as Enoch did. You'll be "on fire" for Christ.

Sing songs of praise and adoration.

Revelation 5:9 says that the saints will sing "a new song" to Jesus. "Sing to the Lord a new song" (Psalm 149:1). What am I doing today? It's extremely hard to sing while I'm frowning, crying, or harboring negative thoughts. People sing when they are happy, celebrating, and being creative. Would it be a blessing to me if I sang to Jesus during my worship time? Children love to sing. Many a mother tells of wheeling through a grocery store with her 2-year-old singing "Jesus Loves Me" at the top of their lungs. Little people have no fear, no hang-ups—they just lift up their voices and sing.

Singing gives power. Singers led the children of Israel around Jericho, and the walls fell down. Singers led armies into battle. Paul and Silas sang in prison while chained to guards. Verse after verse in Psalms tells us to "sing a new song" to the Lord. If you can't carry a tune, don't worry! The Holy Spirit takes our praise to the Father. You can still sing of God's "mercy and justice" (Psalm 101:1).

You're not convinced? Whistle a happy tune. Simply remember: "Let everything that has breath praise the Lord" (Psalm 150:6).

Swallow **your pride.**

The Bible has a lot to say about pride. For starters, "Pride goes before destruction, and a haughty spirit before a fall" (Proverbs 16:18). "Pride will bring him low" (Proverbs 29:23). I'll let you do some studying into this hateful and hurtful way of the heart. Lucifer experienced pride. Paul talks about people being "puffed up" (1 Corinthians 4:18). Others are showier with their prideful ways. Mark describes how Jesus talked of the scribes: "Beware of the scribes, who desire to go around in long robes, love greetings in the marketplaces, the best seats in the synagogues, and the best places at feasts, who devour widows' houses, and for a pretense make long prayers. These will receive greater condemnation" (Mark 12:38-40).What about the rich farmer (fool) whose crop was so large that he boasted that he would "pull down [his] barns and build greater" and take his ease—"eat, drink, and be merry" (Luke 12:18, 19)? He thought he had no needs. First Peter 5:5 says, "God resists the proud, but gives grace to the humble."

Pride isn't just spiritual. We see it in the physical world

as well. Is your marriage in trouble because of your pride? Could you be too proud to say "I'm sorry!" to the husband God has given you? Are you losing your children through pride and faultfinding? Or lashing out at your parents because of this grievous sin? Here's the remedy: "Humble yourselves under the mighty hand of God, that He may exalt you in due time" (1 Peter 5:6).

Speak only the truth in love.

"I always tell the truth!" you say. Congratulations. That's wonderful. And yet, read that line again. You may have missed part of it. Those last two words: "in love." What does "in love" mean? Let me tell you a story you may be able to relate to.

There were some years when, through bad habits and stressful times, I added 30 pounds to my weight. You've probably already guessed: I felt miserable because my clothes were too tight. I looked awful when I looked into the mirror. You get the picture.

One evening, after I spoke to a large group, a woman stopped me. "Honey," she said as she smiled and grabbed my hand, "I haven't seen you for a few years now. You sure did look better when you weren't so fat!"

I responded (after I got over the shock) with "You know, I think you're right."

"Son, tuck in your shirt—you look soooo sloppy."

"Daughter [or sister], with all that makeup you look like a streetwalker. Don't you ever look into a mirror?"

"Friend, you sing loud, but you can't carry a tune in a bucket!"

The truth? Oh, yes. Spoken in love? No, a thousands times no. It's that little member called the tongue. "If anyone among you thinks he is religious, and does not bridle his tongue but deceives his own heart, this one's religion is useless" (James 1:26). Read James 3—the subheading in my Bible calls it "The Untamable Tongue"! The tongue can defile the whole body. Why would I, a daughter of God, discourage one of God's other children with hurtful words? Whenever I'm about to open my mouth, I need to ask myself, "Is this thing I'm about to say for God's glory, or just to get it off my chest? Would I want someone to say this to me?"

We are to bless others, give courage, and show mercy and compassion. Nowhere in the Bible can I find someone exhorting us to "whip anyone into shape." What I do find is that "whatever you want men to do to you, do also to them" (Matthew 7:12).

Chapter Three

THE SUM OF ALL THE PARTS

If We Are What We Eat, We Need Good Food!

Life force. That amazing thing called energy. Do I want to "eat to live," or could it be that I "live to eat"? How long have I been like this? Are the habits I have embraced impossible to overcome? Do I really want to make any changes? What if I went to the doctor and after a checkup and a brief chat was told, "You're killing yourself. You need to make some changes!" Would I change then?

If the physician told me that I looked "pretty good," but I knew that there were many areas in my diet that would not—could not—give me the nutrition my body needed to stay fit, would I then make hard choices and change those destructive habits?

"Good food"——do those two words describe the taste, nutritional value, and freshness of what you and I eat? Perhaps "good" brings to mind that awesome new ice cream that's half price at the supermarket. Sometimes food is "good" because we're eating it in a restaurant that serves very large portions.

Glow with health.

Everywhere I look it seems that a copy of that Food Guide Pyramid looms up before me. Children study it in school. Doctors plaster it on their walls. Nutritionists treat it as their "last will and testament to people everywhere." That's the trouble with health these days: the rules don't go with what's being offered in the supermarkets and restaurants.

Let's put off thinking about those charts for the moment. Here are a few questions to ask yourself: What do I expect from my eating? Will the food I eat make me feel better, more fit, more energetic? Or will my diet pull me down and cause my body to age, to creak and groan under the weight it carries?

You get to choose your diet. Every day! Every meal! No one else can do it for you unless you let go of the reins and drift every which way.

Glory in the knowledge that you are living a life ordained by God.

I know that the Bible says that whatever we eat or drink, we should do it to the glory of God (1 Corinthians 10:31). God paid a price for us and asks us to glorify Him with our bodies (1 Corinthians 6:20). This seems a more serious problem than I first thought. "When I was a child, I spoke as a child, I understood as a child, I thought as a child; but when I became a man, I put away childish things" (1 Corinthians 13:11). Could it be that I have never grown up? *I want what I want! God, don't show me that there is a better way!* "There is a way that seems right to a man, but its end is the way of death" (Proverbs 14:12).

God made a beautiful world and put man and woman in the center. They inherited a perfect garden with every fruit-bearing tree. They were also instructed to enjoy grains and nuts, and later also meat and vegetables. Laws instructed that unclean meats and blood of any kind should be avoided.

What do you and I eat today? What will I choose to place into my body—my temple? "Do you not know that you are the temple of God and that the Spirit of God dwells in you?" (1 Corinthians 3:16).

Give yourself the best nourishment available.

The truth is, when the Food Guide Pyramid suggests

three to five servings of fruits and vegetables a day, it really means we need that many to meet the bare nutritional necessities for health. The best plan includes eight to 10 servings of fruits and vegetables a day.

Whole grains. There are so many. For maximum health we need to search and study—read labels and learn values—until we are familiar with what's really being offered. Do you depend on others to give you directions for your food choices, or do you take responsibility and make *every* effort to consume only foods that will be enriching?

Daniel, along with his three friends, made the hard choices. Dining at the king's table and being so very picky. "None of that meat and wine for me, please. Make it vegetables and water. Vegetables, vegetables, and more vegetables." God blessed their efforts. First, Daniel and his three friends were not put to death. Instead they were given permission to continue eating their strange (to all those around them) diet. Second, at the end of only 10 days everyone could see a difference. The king examined them, and "in all matters of wisdom and understanding about which the king examined them, he found them ten times better than all the magicians and astrologers who were in all his realm" (Daniel 1:20).

Grow through right choices.

What will you place in your basket at the supermarket? When my husband, Dennis, and I decided to make the mind-boggling leap to a completely changed diet, it took the two of us going through refrigerator, freezer, and pantry with garbage bags near at hand. None of this waiting until all the junk food had been consumed. Our bodies were God's temples (and out of control) right now—today! We found, during the process of eliminating junk food and replacing it with fresh healthy food, that once those less-than-healthful foods were no longer available, choosing good things to eat became much easier. Our temptations to cheat were minimal.

Beyond that, when once in a while we do decide to eat a cookie or a "small" dish of ice cream, we find that our tastes have changed. We don't enjoy these treats nearly as much as we used to. Sometimes we can't even finish the longed-for treat.

We had planned to start slowly, but the more healthfully we ate, the better we felt. Suddenly pounds began to melt away. Loose clothes were a reward for our changed behavior. We have no wish to go backward. The biggest question we ask ourselves today is Why did we wait so many years to change our eating habits?

As children grow older, we expect them to make better choices. We encourage them to be more responsible. Can God expect less from you and me?

***Gather* the best information available.**

Begin by gleaning materials from the library. Go to a bookstore and purchase books and magazines that lead you to a better and more healthful diet. Find the most nourishing cookbooks available. Keep in mind, though, that if you go too far too fast, before you are truly ready to stick to your plan, the whole experience may overpower you, and you will give up before you really notice a difference.

Think about slowly replacing some of your old favorite recipes with new healthier ones or reworking them, using more healthful ingredients. It's amazing how little oil you need for frying when you use mostly water with just a small amount of your most healthful oil. Begin to learn how herbs can add to your enjoyment and taste. You may find, as Dennis and I did, that with your more alert taste buds and the addition of healthy seasonings, eating is the best it has ever been.

Look around and find a friend or two with a passion for better eating. Invite your spouse and family to join you as you begin an adventure to slow down your aging and make a difference in the way you look and feel.

Gear up for battle family, friends, and others.

Does this sound a little harsh? Perhaps, but I know how far many of us will go to avoid a fight or even a disagreeable run-in, even if the only alternative is to compromise something we feel strongly about. Here's the kind of situation I'm talking about:

For three days now you've been rocking along on this new eating experience (please, do not think of or call your new way of eating "a diet"). On the fourth day you walk into someone's office and there in front of you is a spread of doughnuts fit for a queen. To go along with this delight are cartons of orange juice, apple juice, and milk. "Help yourself," your friend says. No big deal, you say to yourself. *I'll just take a couple of my favorite doughnuts and a small glass of juice (after all, juice is good for me anyway).*

Let's look again! Thinking *I skipped breakfast anyway; two doughnuts and a small glass of juice will give me a burst of energy* may be the easiest way to handle the situation, but it may also be the worst for your new eating plan. The best choice? Say, "Thanks, but no thanks," then walk quickly away. If you aren't strong enough to walk on, and find yourself standing there with your hand extended, take one doughnut, if you must—then wrap it up and eat it as part of your next meal (but remember to skip the dessert you had already planned to eat!).

An amazing fact to remember: What goes into your

mouth lands somewhere on your body—often as fat. We cannot trick our body into forgiving us a few extra pounds because we were eating with friends or because we just couldn't say no.

The next time you want to slip something extra into your mouth, go to your pantry and pick up a pound of rice. Now, where would you like to place that on your body? Then reach for a five-pound bag of sugar or flour and ask yourself the same question. Is it any wonder that after a few extra "treats" our clothes start feeling tight and refuse to be buttoned?

A week goes by, and a friend slips into your office with an eye-popping slice of cake. "I made it for my special friends. Go ahead; eat up! I made yours extra-large. You're going to love it." The best way to handle the situation? "Thanks, you're so thoughtful. I'll just set it right over here and enjoy it along with my lunch." (At this point, if you are truly serious about what you eat, you may take one or two bites at lunch and unobtrusively throw away the rest. After all, you can wear it or dispose of it. You make the call.) Later in the day you can thank your friend for the wonderful cake.

It may be a mother, sister, husband, wife, coworker, or boss who tempts you to "just try a little." The choice is always up to you. No one can force you to eat or to compromise on your choice of foods. When it seems as though your friend or loved one won't take no for an answer, come back with something like this: "I know my eating so carefully may seem silly/overboard to you, but I find I feel so much better/energetic when I don't eat between meals/overeat/eat sweet things very often." You get the idea. It's not about them—it's about you and being true to what's best for you.

A word of warning: From time to time you will find that

despite all your best efforts, you eat too much or make wrong choices. Now what? My friend and mentor, Bonnie, told me something that puts it all into prospective: "Ginger, if you mess up, go ahead and mess up well. Then forget it and get on with your life. Don't beat yourself up. Pick yourself up, laugh about your pig-out, and begin where you left off before the fateful event."

Gain **a clearer understanding of your body.**

"I will praise You, for I am fearfully and wonderfully made" (Psalm 139:14). The more you learn about your body and the best nutrition you can fill it with, the more you want to eat right.

What tastes better or seems healthier than a large glass of juice: orange, grape, apple, or lemon? Dennis and I found out that most juice can best be described as "high calories and sugar"—never the best choice. How much better for us to eat oranges, apples, a small bunch of grapes, etc.? Suddenly our eyes were opened and we began to understand "a serving." A serving isn't large. *In most cases a serving is a half cup. It's that simple!* So if you want to eat a whole apple, it's two servings. A small banana may be a serving; a large one will probably be two servings.

It's so easy to go from one side of the ditch to the other. First we want to eat everything. Then we choose only the best—but eat enough for three. That's why it's so important to understand our body and its needs. Study for yourself! How much do you need to eat for maximum health?

When you go to that potluck and find tables loaded with wonderful healthy food, you must choose. Eating too much even of good things can only make you feel tired, overfed, and sluggish—not to mention overweight!

If you can't figure out the optimal amount of food for

you and your family, find a nutritionist to work with. Choosing well will not leave you hungry or too full, but feeling satisfied and well fed without that stuffed feeling. A good diet will give you energy and make you feel happy. A poor diet will chip away at your feeling of well-being and cause you to be grouchy and tired.

Grace others with gifts of healthful and healing foods.

Once again this important and well-known verse comes into play: "Whatever you want men to do to you, do also to them" (Matthew 7:12). I can see you smiling. "You're going a bit too far on this one, Ginger. I love to cook, and well, you know, if I ate all the goodies I cooked and baked I'd be as broad as a barn."

Think about it. You decided to make a lifestyle change. You painstakingly went through your pantry, refrigerator, and freezer, leaving only those things that would benefit your body. Six months later and 20 pounds lighter, you feel like a new person.

Suddenly it's your birthday (Independence Day/ Christmas/Easter/whatever anyone wants to celebrate). Will you welcome (or do you need) a bunch of sweets or high-calorie foods?

Let's look at it another way. Suppose you have not changed the way you are living. You are rocking along taking in about 1,000 extra calories a week and slowly outgrowing every stitch of clothes you own. What now? Will a gift of *more calories and sugar* be something to be glad about?

Ask almost anyone, and they'll tell you how much they enjoy these sweet treats—and how much of a temptation or stumbling block they can be. You see, what starts out to be a gift showing how much you really care turns into a gift that will take away the healthy glow from your friend or loved one, not add to it.

What can you do? Again, the key to success is to study. Giving food does not have to mean sabotaging a friend. I like what Matthew writes about gift giving in his Gospel: "What man is there among you who, if his son asks for bread, will give him a stone? Or if he asks for a fish, will he give him a serpent?" (Matthew 7:9, 10).

Do you know how to give good gifts? In the world of overabundance we live in, disposable gifts are great. So are healthy edible ones. Let's see, how about nuts (unsalted/lightly salted)? Natural peanut butter/almond butter? Choice ripe or dried fruit? Gourmet pasta or exotic rice? You take the list from here. In the end you may switch to candles, phone cards, or flowers. Give rein to your creativity and see what you can come up with!

Chapter Four

USE IT OR LOSE IT

Exercise for Health of Body, Mind, and Spirit.

Jane and I met at a women's retreat in a rugged and beautiful mountain setting. I couldn't help feeling an eagerness to walk some of the trails visible from the rooms where we were staying. Coming from a different time zone, I rose early that first morning and began my adventure as quickly as possible.

That's when I met Jane. While most of the other women slept, her passion for exercise had brought her also to the early-morning trails. Together we enjoyed not only a brisk climb but also an opportunity to get to know each other.

A short way into our walk I knew I'd have to put all the energy I could muster into keeping up with Jane. I noticed also that she walked with a slight limp that became more pronounced as we went along.

"Is your leg hurting¿" I asked solicitously.

"No more than usual," she replied.

"There must be a story here." I mused. I listened horrified and amazed as she told a tale of filling her car with gasoline. The task didn't take much thought, and she had almost completed it when the accident happened. An older man became confused as he prepared to leave the gas station. As he put his car into gear and pressed his foot to the gas pedal, he made a serious mistake. He chose "drive" instead of "reverse."

Seconds later Jane lay in agony with one leg almost severed just above the knee. After many hours of grueling surgery, the doctors warned her that she would never be able to walk again without crutches. Gone were her days of exploring the mountain trails and freedom of movement.

"I couldn't accept that verdict." she continued. "My first walk around this beautiful lake, taken months after the accident, remains a vivid memory. Tears fell freely as I took one agonizing step after another, over boulders and through washes—on my crutches. I couldn't give up. I wouldn't give up!"

That day I learned something about the human spirit. We all need vision, and each of us gets to decide what condition each day will find us in. Oh, yes, horrible things can happen, circumstances can take away our ability for a time or a lifetime. How we react and whether we continue as normally as possible are both up to us. Hard work brings a lifetime of rewards. If we sit down and give up, we will lose even the limited amount of stamina and mobility that remains in us.

Think of such expressions as "couch potato," "veg out," "take a break." What pictures come to your mind? Inactivity? Laziness? King Solomon, the wisest man who ever lived, said, "Laziness casts one into a deep sleep, and an idle person will suffer hunger" (Proverbs 19:15). Then he goes on to say, "A lazy man buries his hand in the bowl, and will not so much as bring it to his mouth again" (verse 24). A pretty sorry portrait if he's describing us.

"Moses was one hundred and twenty years old when he died. His eyes were not dim nor his natural vigor diminished" (Deuteronomy 34:7). Could that be describing you or me in our 30s, 40s, 50s, or even 70s?

Less than six months ago and 30 pounds heavier, I would often invite my husband, Dennis, to take a walk with me. I would promise him that we didn't have to go too far—hoping for a mile. The ensuing walk, if he choose to accompany me, would usually be less than a block and often at a snail's pace. *He just doesn't get it!* I'd think.

Then came that memorable day when together we chose to make deliberate and incredible life changes. Suddenly Dennis started asking *me* to walk with *him*. We settled on a route that took us to the highway and back along our dead-end road, more than two miles. On pretty days, or at times when we felt unhurried, we would even stretch our walk to three miles. Soon came lovely weekends when our three-mile walks extended to five miles, and eventually to nine miles.

Did we always feel like walking? Certainly not! We chose to walk—in the dark, in the fog and mist, even in the cold. Sometimes after an evening walk morning came all too soon—but out we went again.

The difference came gradually. Ten pounds. Twenty. Thirty, and still they dropped. He lost two for each one of mine! But more than pounds, we lost inches. We learned that muscle weighs more than fat. Therefore, we watched and celebrated the loss of inches more than pounds.

Were there any down sides? Some—but too few to mention. When your jeans literally fall off your hips, the laughter you share seems priceless. Trips to Goodwill with our outgrown wardrobe became weekly celebrations. Overcrowded closets filled with no-longer-wearable clothing soon began to feel roomy and inviting.

Take a few suggestions from those who have walked before:

Enter **into a pact with God.**

The apostle Paul shares a promise I couldn't live without . . . wouldn't want to live without: "And He [God] said to me [Paul], 'My grace is sufficient for you, for My strength is made perfect in weakness.' Therefore most gladly I will rather boast in my infirmities, that the power of Christ may rest upon me. . . . For when I am weak, then I am strong" (2 Corinthians 12:9, 10). Now read it again, placing your name where Paul's is.

Can you believe it? You don't need superpower to walk the walk. You need Christ. You need to surrender yourself and your life to Him and take just one step at a time. Need more encouragement? Read Psalm 18:32, 33: "It is God who arms me with strength, and makes my way perfect. He makes my feet like the feet of deer, and sets me on my high places." What a promise!

The rewards of this contract with God are something else. They bring us to the next step.

Endure the pain, but feel the gain.

Health experts tell us that we should not do so much exercise that we are left hurting. That's easy for them to say—you and I are on a mission and find stopping before pain a difficult task. Be careful, of course, but don't avoid your daily walk because you feel stiff and a bit sore. Too often those things are just an excuse to miss "a day or two" of exercise.

Set goals and stick to them. Most books and magazines suggest that you get in at least 30 minutes of exercise five times a week. Keep in mind that this suggestion is the bare minimum—the least you can do and squeak through calling yourself "in shape."

The main thing to ask yourself: What are my expectations for exercise? Do I expect just to realize minimal goals or am I intent on feeling a difference? Can I do more than "just enough" to avoid the inactive label? Dennis and I have found that success begets success, and we keep aiming higher. We find that the older we get, the greater our need to keep active and fit.

How serious do you think this admonition is in Hebrews 12:1? "Since we are surrounded by so great a cloud of witnesses, let us lay aside every weight, and the sin which so easily ensnares us, and let us run with endurance the race that is set before us."

Isaiah tell us, "Those who wait on the Lord shall renew their strength; they shall mount up wings like eagles, they shall run and not be weary, they shall walk and not faint" (Isaiah 40:31). If that will be our state in heaven, doesn't it seem to you that we should begin practicing here and now?

Experience the glow.

Have you ever run across a happy person? A woman, a man, or a child filled with cheerfulness, a caring spirit, the energy and love of God? They stand out. Others want to know what makes that person happy, with the hope that some of their joy will rub off.

King David talks a lot about happiness. One of my favorite statements is "Happy are the people whose God is the Lord!" (Psalm 144:15).

We can have that happiness from God in good times, at times when life seems unmanageable—and even when life's whirling us about in times of sorrow and suffering. How often have you asked the question that David asked in a time of distress, "Why are you cast down, O my soul? And why are you disquieted within me? Hope in God; for I shall yet praise Him, the help of my countenance and my God" (Psalm 42:11).

Can not we expect the same blessing that God asked Moses to share with Aaron and his sons so they could then bless the children of Israel? "The Lord bless you and keep you; the Lord make His face shine upon you, and be gracious to you; the Lord lift up His countenance upon you, and give you peace" (Numbers 6:24-26). A shining face reflecting God's blessing—that's what I want. Some refer to it as "the glow of health—another one of God's blessings." When you and I have this remarkable gift, we find ourselves energetic and hardly out of breath when others are panting and have already given up and are unable to walk another step.

But we must go on. What else should we look forward

to each day?

Enjoy the company of God and others.

If you haven't done so already, embark today on a life-long study to understand what it means to be a friend of God's. When you have immersed yourself completely in the Bible and God's gift of love, you will find that this friendship, this love, is deep enough to be studied throughout the ages.

Does God reluctantly accept you as a friend when you finally come crawling on hands and knees begging for forgiveness and His blessing? Is He a stranger who already has enough friends and hasn't got time for you? Consider His words in John 15:9: "As the Father loved Me, I also have loved you; abide in My love."

So the real question is not whether God loves me and wants to be my friend, but How do I find God? Friendship must be active. It's not one-sided. God's assurance to the children of Israel, when they found themselves scattered and far from Him, still stands today: "You will seek the Lord your God, and you will find Him if you seek Him with all your heart and with all your soul" (Deuteronomy 4:29).

The promises in the Bible to those who seek God are wonderful. In Isaiah 55:1-6 come these familiar words: "Ho! Everyone who thirsts, come to the waters. . . . And let your soul delight itself in abundance. Incline your ear, and come to Me. Hear, and your soul shall live; and I will make an everlasting covenant with you. . . . Seek the Lord while He may be found, call upon Him while He is near."

Now go back and read the whole chapter. You'll read about people who don't know God is running to *them*. God promises mercy and pardon. He talks about accomplishing and prospering. Finding joy and peace. Singing and clapping.

The idea seems too wonderful to imagine. A true friend

who will never leave us or forsake us (Hebrews 13:5). "You will seek Me and find Me, when you search for Me with all your heart" (Jeremiah 29:13).

Then what?

Then you will understand the value of a true friend. Friendship comes to us on this earth in so many ways. When we are small, our mother and father fulfill all our desires for companionship. As we get older, we want more. Brothers and sisters share our lives. Grandparents, aunts, uncles, and cousins enlarge our world. Husbands and wives, business partners and coworkers, neighbors and others we encounter on life's journey: all bring strength and learning into our lives.

King Solomon summed it up this way: "Two are better than one, because they have a good reward for their labor. For if they fall, one will lift up his companion. But woe to him who is alone when he falls, for he has no one to help him up. Again, if two lie down together, they will keep warm; but how can one be warm alone? Though one may be overpowered by another, two can withstand him. And a threefold cord is not quickly broken" (Ecclesiastes 4:9-12).

About marriage God said "It is not good that man should be alone" (Genesis 2:18) and "A man shall leave his father and mother and be joined to his wife, and they shall become one" (Genesis 2:24). We find the disciples going out in twos (Luke 10:1), as did others with a mission, such as Moses and Aaron, Paul and Silas.

Last, I invite you to turn to the counsel from the wisest man who ever lived. It'll make you a much sought-after friend, and it's found in Proverbs 17:22: "A merry heart [some call it laughter] does good, like medicine." Or in the Message translation: "A cheerful disposition is good for your health." Keeping a smile on your face is exercising the muscles that make a difference to yourself and others you come in contact with.

Escape and enjoy a taste of heaven.

"Escape what?" you ask. "I'm a busy person. I have meals to fix, children to raise, a job to go to—and this is just the beginning of my day's work."

You're correct. I have no argument with you there. When God put man and woman in the garden, He gave them work to do (Genesis 2:15-22). Read the Bible from Genesis to Revelation and you will find that work has been a part of people's lives throughout history. Work is not the problem. It keeps us strong, healthy, and focused. We run into trouble when we make work our only goal.

In the Garden of Eden, God walked and talked with Adam and Eve in the evening. Jesus went to the garden to be with His father and to draw strength and courage for the days ahead. David, in talking about God as our refuge, quotes Him this way: "Be still, and know that I am God; I will be exalted among the nations, I will be exalted in the earth! The Lord of hosts is with us; the God of Jacob is our refuge" (Psalm 46:10, 11).

Life is not about us. It's about us being right with God. How can we have a relationship if we spend no time with Him? If our homes are to be a little taste of heaven on earth, we must give God time in our homes every day.

Jesus says, "Come." "If anyone thirsts, let him come to Me and drink" (John 7:37). "Come to Me, all you who labor and are heavy laden, and I will give you rest" (Matthew 11:28).

We must turn toward Him. Take a step forward. Listen! Be still. It doesn't matter when or where. God wants to commune with us and give us abundant blessings. Perhaps more than we have room enough to receive.

How will you escape the hustle and bustle of everyday living? Use your imagination. Get up a little earlier than the others. Study and pray after your family has gone to bed. Study with those around you. Make a prayer closet, a prayer room, take a prayer walk and commune with God in the beauty of nature.

What will you do when you come to God? You can take Him your fears (Psalm 27:1; Isaiah 35:4; Luke 12:32; 2 Timothy 1:7; 1 John 4:18), hand over your burdens (Psalm 55:22; Matthew 11:30), and talk about your enemies (Psalm 18:48; 23:5; 25:2; 119:98; Matthew 5:44; Luke 1:71). Sing, pray, talk, walk—you can even whistle! At times you will weep and cry, beg and plead, humble yourself, and express joy unlimited. You don't even need to do anything. Just listen, be still and know, take deep breaths and run toward God. He'll do the rest.

Expect results from yielding to God.

You may have seen the story on the Internet about a little teacup that gets very angry when its maker throws it on the potter's wheel and forces it into shape, then fires it in a hot kiln, glazes it, and fires it again. All those things *hurt!* But it emerges happy with its beautiful shape and smooth, flawless design. (See Appendix B.)

The story of the little teacup is a wonderful analogy of our lives. Smooth? At times. On the other hand, sometimes it seems as if the people who have the deepest relationship with God are the ones who face the most trials. But if we get on our knees when the heat becomes overwhelming, God knows and cares. He says, "Count it all joy" (James 1:2).

When you were a child and went to school, you studied and learned. It's the same when you go to God. "Take my yoke upon you and learn from Me" (Matthew 11:29). A moment with God can be wasted only if we do not pay attention. God, who is good, teaches us His goodness. We see our life through different eyes. We no longer love sin—any sin—but we love the sinner through Him, the one who made each one of us in His own image.

Seeing our life through God's eyes of love gives us a different picture. Speaking of God's everlasting love, Paul shows us that no matter what happens to us, "in all these things we are more than conquerors through Him who loved us," because nothing can separate us "from the love of God which is in Christ Jesus our Lord" (Romans 8:37, 39).

Effect a change in yourself and others.

Changed. Different. Not the same as before. When you have exercised and grown through your relationship with Christ, nothing is ever the same again. That's what change is like.

Some of my favorite Bible characters found this to be true. Jacob wrestled with God. What a night! Who won? They both won, but Jacob's name was changed to Israel to represent the new man he became that night. Saul became Paul, more ardent to bring men and women to God than he had been to destroy them only days earlier. Philip, doing God's bidding, in a short time changed the Ethiopian's life.

Job went through every stage of crisis and loss. He became angry and arrogant. He listened to and reproached his close friends. He even disagreed with his wife and refused to curse God and die. As He gave up and listened to God, Job finally said, "Behold, I am vile; What shall I answer You? I lay my hand over my mouth. Once I have spoken, but I will not answer; yes, twice, but I will proceed no further" (Job 40:4, 5). He began to learn one of life's hard lessons. Read Job's reply to God in repentance and experience his restoration in Job 42.

Jonah watched God change a whole city when it was confronted with its wickedness. Read his story. Listen to the people and king of Nineveh after every man, woman, and child has repented in sackcloth and ashes: "Who can tell if God will turn and relent, and turn away from His fierce anger, so that we many not perish?" (Jonah 3:9) Result? "Then God saw their works, that they turned from their evil way; and God relented from the disaster that He had said He would bring upon them, and He did not do it" (verse 10).

Embark on an energized life.

My favorite hymn of faith comes from Habakkuk. The prophet had a burden. He wasn't sure why he could not see God acting on his behalf. He questioned God. He listened to God. Yet I find that I want to pray the very words that come at the end of his prayer in Habakkuk 3:17-19:

> "Though the fig tree may not blossom,
> Nor fruit be on the vines;
> Though the labor of the olive may fail,
> And the fields yield no food;
> Though the flock be cut off from the fold,
> And there be no herd in the stalls—
> Yet I will rejoice in the Lord,
> I will joy in the God of my salvation.
> The Lord God is my strength;
> He will make my feet like deer's feet,
> And He will make me walk on my high hills."

Chapter Five

YOU CAN'T LIVE WITHOUT IT!

Water—for Life and Healing

"What's that you say I can't live without?" you ask. "Could you be talking about the staff of life—you know, bread? Or perhaps you're planning to take a look at a favorite food of so many people—potatoes? If not these, where are you going next?"

Some might think they can't live without television, motorcycles, and fast cars, or even family and friends. These things all seem to find a place in our world today. Yet none of them hold a candle to this next law of health.

Which of the above-mentioned objects make up about two thirds of our bodies and 85 percent of our brains? Aha, now you can see we're getting serious. It could well be the difference between life and death. You see, there are only a few things we can go without for a shorter period of time. Why would you not embrace it? Try to list the different forms and uses there are for it and you'll understand all the more the importance of this fifth need of the human body. Drink it, bathe in it, use it for recreation. But that's not all. Without this wonderful element, grass would turn brown and die. Trees would cease to grow their leaves and wither away. There would be no vegetable gardens or flowers to brighten the landscape and bring nourishment to each of us. Enough said. You know, of course, that we're talking about *water*.

There would be no quality of life without water. In fact, life could be sustained for only a short period without it, even if the weather were cool and you did nothing but sit in quiet reverie in the shade.

Some suggest that we probably get enough water in our daily diets. These folks say, "Live any way you want. Don't worry or fret about getting enough water." Others strongly suggest that we drink *at least* eight 8-ounce glasses of pure water a day.

Think about cooking a pot of potatoes. You know from experience that they need at least six cups of water to cook properly. Will you skimp and add only three cups, hoping that the potatoes will not burn? Will you experiment to see if perhaps as few as two cups will do the job or only scorch them a little? You might be more apt to add an extra cup to be sure, and also to take care of any problem that might occur if you got back to them a few minutes late.

The same goes for your body. Are you serving yourself best if you skimp on your water intake? How can you ask God to heal all your diseases (Psalm 103:3) if you don't even care enough to do the things you know can make a difference?

Healing is found in each of the eight steps below that go along with water, which we value for its healing and life-sustaining properties. Let me show you what I mean:

Whisper a prayer.

The way a prayer ascends to the Father makes no difference. You can shout, breathe, or whisper a prayer and the end product will still be the same. God tells us to "watch and pray" (Matthew 26:41); "pray without ceasing" (1 Thessalonians 5:17); "pray and not lose heart" (Luke 18:1).

We "watch and pray" lest we fall into temptation. As a parent you will go to almost any length to keep your children from temptation and its harmful effects. God feels the same way about us. That's why He has sent the Holy Spirit to interpret our groanings. "The Spirit also helps in our weaknesses. For we do not know what we should pray for as we ought, but the Spirit Himself makes intercession for us with groanings which cannot be uttered. Now He who searches the hearts knows what the mind of the Spirit is, because He makes intercession for the saints according to the will of God" (Romans 8:26, 27).

Daniel found that praying in a certain place at a certain time kept him connected to God. These were times that he could pour out his heart in thanks and supplication before his God (Daniel 6:10, 11). Daniel also determined in his heart that nobody, not even the king, could sway him from worship and prayer.

How long has it been since you and I made such a commitment to the One who gives us life? Would we be willing to give our all just for one more chance to connect with Heaven?

The "whys" of our prayers make no difference. We can ask for a clean heart, salvation, faith, healing, or just cry out in pain and misery with the assurance that the God who created you and me "heals the brokenhearted and binds up their wounds" (Psalm 147:3).

Will a lifetime be long enough to study the effect that prayer has on us? What about on our families and those we love? For whom do you pray? Can you, knowing that the devil goes forth as a roaring lion (1 Peter 5:8), afford to limit your times of prayer—or perhaps even skip any or all of your opportunities to commune with God?

The next step tries me and often seems impossible to accomplish.

Wait on the Lord.

Wait? You've got to be kidding. I'm too busy! You're telling me that God instructs me to "wait" (Psalm 27:14)?

Yes. Think about this: You've just gotten out of your car and now, as you wait to cross the street, the traffic seems heavier than usual. What will you do next: (a) wait for the traffic to clear and proceed across the street when it is safe? (b) cross the street in front of the traffic and hope all of the oncoming cars will stop? (c) say a prayer and walk boldly across, expecting God to protect you? (d) get back into your car and drive away discouraged, because crossing seems impossible?

Or look at it another way: The doctor enters the room with a grin from one ear to the other. "I've got great news," he almost shouts. "Your twins will be delivered in a little less than seven months."

I can just hear your curt reply. "What do you mean 'seven months,' doctor? My husband and I refuse to listen to that kind of talk. We want our babies, and we want them now!"

Would what you want make a difference? Nature must take its course. In matters of life we have come to expect and accept the inconveniences of waiting. Yet with God, we want an immediate answer. Does it remind you of the saying, "Lord, give me patience, and give it to me *now!*"

David had it right when he wrote,

> "I waited patiently for the Lord;
> And He inclined to me,
> And heard my cry.
> He also brought me up out of a horrible pit,
> Out of the miry clay,
> And set my feet upon a rock,
> And established my steps.
> He has put a new song in my mouth—
> Praise to our God;
> Many will see it and fear,
> And will trust in the Lord" (Psalm 40:1-3).

Wrestle with jealousy and faultfinding.

Can you find any good in the word "jealous"? Would you be happy if your friends, family, or coworkers described you as "green with envy"? I dare say you would deny all allegations of jealousy and do everything within your power to prove those words false.

So why do I find myself so often looking at things that my friend has been blessed with? Is it an accident when the tenth commandment says, "You shall not covet your neighbor's house; you shall not covet your neighbor's wife, nor his male servant, nor his female servant, nor his ox, nor his donkey, nor *anything* that is your neighbor's" (Exodus 20:17)?

That commandment seems quite clear. Instead of wishing I had what belongs to another, I'm instructed by God to "consider the lilies of the field" (Matthew 6:28) and the "birds of the air" (verse 26), to "not worry about tomorrow" (verse 34).

The practical wisdom Solomon shares goes this way, "Consider the work of God; for who can make straight what He has made crooked? In the day of prosperity be joyful, but in the day of adversity consider: surely God has appointed the one as well as the other, so that man can find out nothing that will come after him" (Ecclesiastes 7:13, 14).

Do you remember the saying we often repeated as kids, "Sticks and stones may break my bones, but words can't hurt my body"? As adults we realize how silly that saying really was. Words wound!

You and I get to choose. We can live the life of Psalm 19:14, "Let the words of my mouth and the mediation of my heart be acceptable in Your sight, O Lord, my strength and my Redeemer." Or we can follow the easy and sinful course of Proverbs 10:14, "The mouth of the foolish is near destruction."

Solomon goes on to say, "A lying tongue hates those

who are crushed by it, and a flattering mouth works ruin" (Proverbs 26:28).

A lying tongue—who will it harm the most, me or those I use it against? Study Romans 12:9-21. How does a Christian behave? As I said, we get to choose.

Weep for yourself and others.

Imagine a world in which there is no sin and evil. A world where the little child will lead the wild animals and play by the cobra's hole (Isaiah 11:6-8). But these words do not describe our world. It's in heaven that there will be no more crying.

In this world of sin and sorrow we need to be available to others. "As one whom his mother comforts, so I will comfort you," God says to us (Isaiah 66:13). "Can a woman forget her nursing child, and not have compassion on the son of her womb?" And sadly, He has to answer, "Surely [she] may forget" (Isaiah 49:15).

You and I can be different. We *must* be different. As Paul describes a Christian in Romans 12 he says this, "Bless those who persecute you; bless and do not curse. Rejoice with those who rejoice, and weep with those who weep" (verses 14, 15).

Death is part of life on this earth. Eccelesiastes 9:5 announces the grim news: "The living know that they will die." That knowledge gives us an edge. Instead of fearing sorrow and death, we have hope in the coming of the Lord. That hope will enable you and me to be God's hands—hands with flesh on them.

Who will be there for the young mother who suffers a miscarriage? Will someone extend a strong shoulder to the parent or spouse who looses one they love to suicide? When disease and sickness strikes you or one you care about, the touch of another person who has walked the road or a friend with a strong faith will see you through.

"Weeping may endure for a night, but joy comes in the morning" (Psalm 30:5). How can I be part of that joy? I am so thankful that God equipped men and women with tears. What a wonderful way to wash away the awfulness of sin and suffering. Where would we be if no crying were allowed? "Rejoice with those who rejoice, and weep with those who weep." It's the highest form of caring.

Wonder "why"; it's an OK question.

Sometimes as a parent or teacher we respond to "Why?" with "Because I said so!" It's expected to be the end of the discussion. What about our heavenly Father? Does He cut us short and expect every evil thing to be taken without a murmur? Consider the familiar Bible heroes whose stories you have read and reread during your lifetime. How often have they been bold enough to question God's leading? Most surprisingly, they often received an answer to their question. Yet not in every circumstance.

John the Baptist, from his prison cell, sent a straightforward message to Jesus: "Are You the Coming One, or do we look for another?" (Luke 7:20). Jesus understood why John had asked the question and responded plainly, telling John's disciples to go and report all they had seen and heard.

Mary and Martha both asked, "Lord, if you had only been here!" (see John 11:20, 21, 32). I can imagine they had seen Jesus heal the sick and at least heard stories of the dead He had raised. Still, in their hour of need, "Why?" was an appropriate first question to ask.

It's OK to ask "Why?" But don't dwell there. Move on.

Wish for "when," but live "while."

Following close on the heels of "Why?" you often find

the question "When?" The disciples expected Jesus to set up His kingdom here on earth. What a disappointment when during the triumphal entry Jesus didn't work a miracle. How easy it would have been for Him to take over the government with all that support. How could they understand when He was arrested and refused to fight back? "When will Your promised kingdom be set up, Lord?" remained the all-consuming question. They didn't understand! They had been with Him so long and yet they seemed to have no clue.

The well-loved gospel hymn says it best: "Have Thine own way, Lord! Have Thine own way!" It ends with "While I am waiting, yielded and still." It's so hard to wait. Place yourself in the army of Israelites waiting to cross the Red Sea. Picture Moses asking God, "Why did You bring us to this dead end? When will You make Your way known? Even I know that this is a bad situation."

Instead of being angry and retaliating, God ignores the "when" and goes on with the "while" of opening up the dry path. I see His "while" in turning salty water to sweet, in making an ax-head float. He acts while others fear the outcome of David's encounter with Goliath, and invites Peter to join him while the disciples shake from fear on a stormy sea.

Jesus says it best in the awesome passage (Luke 12:26-32) in which He tells us not to worry. He begins, "If you then are not able to do the least, why are you anxious for the rest?" and closes by reminding us, "Do not fear, little flock, for it is your Father's good pleasure to give you the kingdom."

Walk with God at all times.

Where do you and I find healing? Where can we go for rest? Who can heal my troubled heart? Who cares about me? These and many questions like them have been asked through the ages.

The Bible overflows with stories of people who needed healing. And a common thread runs through them all: Jesus is the great healer! To those who were blind or had leprosy, to those running from the threat of death or from a storm that threatens to overcome them, Jesus was the one who stretched out His arm to heal and calm the storms. Study the Gospels. Jesus walks with us, talks with us, and heals us.

He's also the one who gives us rest. I love the old hymn that says, "There is a place of quiet rest, near to the heart of God." When we come to Him with all our burdens, we will find rest for our souls.

How often do you find yourself or those you love suffering from a troubled heart? Turn to God: "Let not your heart be troubled; you believe in God, believe also in Me. In My Father's house are many mansions; if it were not so, I would have told you. I go to prepare a place for you" (John 14:1, 2). How tenderly Jesus responds to His troubled children.

Martha couldn't understand. Mary seemed once again bent on letting her down. The time had come to confront the offender head-on. But she didn't reckon with her Lord. "Jesus answered and said to her, 'Martha, Martha, you are worried and troubled about many things. But one thing is needed, and Mary has chosen that good part, which will not be taken away from her'" (Luke 10:41, 42).

Who cares when your heart breaks? Listen as Peter invites you to turn to Jesus: "Casting all your care upon Him, for He cares for you" (1 Peter 5:7).

Write **of God's love and watchcare.**

Think of the times you or somebody you know about has received God's wonderful gift of healing. How do you remember these events? Do you think of them often? Do you tell others?

God's love cannot be contained in any one person, but we can share with others what we've seen and experienced. What about keeping a journal of God's care over you and your family? Would writing of the day's events bring you new awareness and faith? Would your story be a blessing to others? We can write it in our hearts. We can place it in the minds of our friends and families by telling each exciting story of healing and deliverance. We can keep it fresh by giving thanks to God in our prayers and songs of praise. We can write it and share it in paper and ink.

Once again we must be careful what words we use. We can say, "I was sure lucky today. I left my purse on in the busy restaurant, and someone turned it in to the front desk." Or we can say "How blessed I was today. Instead of tears of sorrow over a lost purse when I forgot it during our lunch, I am so grateful to God because someone chose to turn it in to the front desk!"

"I did it all myself," or "Praise the Lord." You get the picture.

Chapter Six

"IF ONLY I HAD THE TIME!"

Rest Is One of God's Commands.

It's been one of those days. You got up early thinking of a million (give or take a few) things that had to be done before your head hits the pillow again. Little did you know how far off track you'd be before the morning ended. A dead battery, a sick child, an overflowing sink, and a neighbor in need all took a portion of your precious morning hours. Now you find yourself facing the afternoon in more of a panic than you thought possible. In the haste of the hour, you've made matters worse by locking yourself out of the house. Feelings of "woe is me" fill your soul.

Back up. Let's look at the picture again. How many of those "must do's" were really only "want to do's"? Which things on the long list of "do before sunset and sleep" were only your attempt at being superwoman? What if some of the things on the list you so carefully assembled earlier don't get done today, tomorrow, or even this week? Will you survive? Will the sun keep shining and the birds continue singing?

It's time to remember the things that are important in our lives. This brings us to law number six—rest—and causes us to reevaluate our lives once again. Ask yourself this question: *Will what I am doing or planning to do today be worth cutting my life short for?* No matter what answer you give, read on. What you find may surprise you, or it may just give you peace of mind.

I can just hear you thinking, *Ginger, you have to be kidding! How can you expect a busy person like me to take "time out," so to speak? Isn't that for naughty children, the young, and perhaps the old? I have places to go and things to do before I sleep. Give me a break!* OK, let's look at rest in a few different ways.

Remember the Sabbath day.

We first run into "resting" in Genesis 2:2, 3: "On the seventh day God ended His work which He had done, and He rested on the seventh day from all His work which He had done. Then God blessed the seventh day and sanctified it, because in it He rested from all His work which God had created and made."

It's hard to be any plainer than that. God Himself planned for us to rest and rested Himself. Am I busier than God was in creating a world? *Perhaps not. . . . OK, I'm definitely not!*

Let's skip ahead to Exodus 20:8-11. You can probably recite these verses from memory. Yet at times you and I both forget what they really mean: "Remember the Sabbath day, to keep it holy. Six days you shall labor and do all your work, but the seventh day is the Sabbath of the Lord your God. In it you shall do no work: you, nor your son, nor your daughter, nor your male servant, nor your female servant, nor your cattle, nor your stranger who is within your gates. For in six days the Lord made the heavens and the earth, the sea, and all that is in them, and rested the seventh day. Therefore the Lord blessed the Sabbath day and hallowed it."

We know God rested. He also asked us to hallow His Sabbaths, "to bring no burden through the gates of this city on the Sabbath day, but hallow the Sabbath day, to do no work in it" (Jeremiah 17:24). It seems quite plain what He wants from us. As we study the Gospels, we find that Jesus went to the synagogue and kept the Sabbath that He had made for human beings (Luke 4:15; Mark 2:27).

***Raise* an altar of thanksgiving and remembrance.**

After the Flood "Noah built an altar to the Lord, and
took of every clean animal and of every clean bird, and offered burnt offerings on the altar" (Genesis 8:20). Study the
life of Abraham. He often built altars to God (Genesis 12:6-
9; 13:18). I'm fascinated by the account of the tribe of
Reuben, the tribe of Gad, and the half the tribe of Manasseh
in the book of Joshua. "Therefore we said, 'Let us now prepare to build ourselves an altar, not for burnt offering nor
for sacrifice, but that it may be a witness between you and
us and our generations after us, . . . that your descendants
may not say to our descendants in time to come, 'You have
no part in the Lord.' Therefore we said that it will be, when
they say this to us or to our generations in time to come,
that we may say, 'Here is the replica of the altar of the Lord
which our fathers made, though not for burnt offerings nor
for sacrifices; but it is a witness between you and us'"
(Joshua 22:26-28).

What am I building between God and my family "as a
witness between God and us"? Is it important for us to place
God in the center of the special times of our lives?

God gave the greatest commandment to the children of
Israel: "Hear, O Israel: The Lord our God, the Lord is one! You
shall love the Lord your God with all your heart, with all your
soul, and with all your strength. . . . You shall teach [these
words] diligently to your children, and shall talk of them
when you sit in your house, when you walk by the way,
when you lie down, and when you rise up. You shall bind
them as a sign on your hand, and they shall be as frontlets between your eyes. You shall write them on the doorposts of
your house and on your gates" (Deuteronomy 6:4-9).

Again God has spelled it out. It really is important to
keep God's love and goodness to His children *forever* (from

the beginning of time as well as through our lifetime) as the center or theme of our homes.

Read, read, read.

Someone has said, "If you or I aren't growing, then we are shrinking—the mind does not stay in neutral."

What would God have me to do when He asks me to "study to shew [myself] approved unto God" (2 Timothy 2:15, KJV)? I like to think that God has provided the Holy Scriptures as our first guidebook, our most important place to channel our learning. If I faithfully avail myself of the wisdom therein, I can and will become a new person, a new creature.

I have found that there are many things in nature that also expand my horizon and teach me of God's ways. These lessons, one of which is the habits of ants, can be learned in a few minutes or over days, months, and years. Reading nature, the seasons, and the characteristics of God's children open my mind still further.

God has given each of us a clear mind to discern the best things for our body. What will you put into your mind? Will it be possible to live successfully in and adapt to the world around us if we do not have a sense of history, science, and the arts? Unless we have endless time, energy, and funds for traveling, our lives can be enriched by studying about other areas of our world, other people's ways of doing things, and perhaps better ways to relate to these people.

How important will I find it to make a study of the human body, what it needs to stay in top shape, and the importance of choosing my diet wisely? Am I educated in these matters enough to make lifelong decisions for myself and my family?

Take a minute and respond to the following questions: How do I feel about a physician who doesn't read? Can my pastor hold my attention each week if he or she never opens a book or magazine? Do I expect those who teach my children to continue to develop their minds through the written and spoken word?

While reading can rest and relax your body, it's also a great way to expand your mind.

Refer to God's wonderful deeds to His children.

Whom can I talk to? What should I talk about? If I make God central in my life and the things I talk about, will those around me enjoy my company or sigh with relief when I depart? These are serious questions.

The Bible says, "When I was a child, I spoke as a child, I understood as a child, I thought as a child; but when I became a man, I put away childish things" (1 Corinthians 13:11). Children prattle on, whether or not anyone shows any interest in what they are saying or even is listening at all. As we grow older and wiser we can discern interest and read the body language of others. Suddenly our eyes are opened, and we experience an awakening and perhaps a change in our habits of communicating.

When God instructed Philip to go to a certain road and speak to a man, Philip first asked the eunuch if he wanted help in understanding the scripture he was reading. More than that, he then waited for an answer and an invitation before stepping into the chariot. On the other hand, Stephen spoke openly to a crowd of angry and treacherous leaders and was stoned. So how are we to determine the style and extent of our sharing?

I remember slipping out early one morning while attending a camp meeting to take a brisk walk. I ignored the light mist and began following the winding sidewalks around the campus where I was staying. Quite a way from my dorm, I met a man jogging toward me. He slowed slightly as we met, and I offered him a cheery "Good morning!" He nodded his head, but the memorable part of his response came after he had passed. In an unmistakable voice loud enough for me to hear he declared, "I surely do love Jesus." Wow! What a witness those few words have been to me.

The older I get and the longer I live on this world, I am persuaded that we want to share only when we have something meaningful to talk about. The more we fall in love with our Savior, the easier it gets. What about you? Will you speak of Him often, or remain silent and let another tell of the good things that come with having Jesus as the center of one's life?

Relax: **Take plenty of time for sleep and rest.**

It has been many years now, but the memory of that night remains fresh in my mind. I had been a friend of Joy's* for almost a year. Her life had been hard. Although she had lost quite a bit of weight, she had much more to lose. Her older daughter had been raped, and the little one swore almost every time she opened her mouth. Joy's common-law husband stayed away from home almost as much as he was there.

The shock of the phone's shrill ring woke Dennis and me with a feeling of dread. *Who could be calling at this hour?* raced through both of our minds.

My "Hello" was met with a teary voice on the other end.

"Ginger, you *have* to come and get my daughters, *quickly!*"

"Wait! Am I talking to Joy?"

"Yes. . . . Please come quickly, Ginger. I can't sleep anymore." Sobs filled my ear. "I'm going to kill myself. Please come and take the girls."

Sleep fled from me in that instant. "I've got to go!" I

stammered to Dennis. "Joy says she plans to kill herself. I have to hurry . . ." Already my feet had hit the floor, and I rushed toward the closet.

Dennis followed close behind. "We'll both go," he responded.

We found Joy sobbing. Beside herself with weariness, she had gone beyond the point of reason. For a few moments I just held her. Then I pulled away and gently suggested we talk as Dennis sat quietly across the room.

"It's hopeless, Ginger. I can't sleep anymore. I know if I close my eyes I will never wake up again, and I can't keep going any longer." Sobs came again, and I waited.

What was the story behind Joy's fear, grief, and breakdown? A friend sharing a "truth" (as she saw it) had convinced Joy that God required Joy's death so that Joy's common-law husband could become a decent man and be saved.

I've always been grateful that the Holy Spirit impressed us to bring a Bible along that night. I opened its pages to the promise that Joy needed most, found in Psalm 4:8: "I will both lie down in peace, and sleep; for You alone, O Lord, make me dwell in safety."

So many demons chased Joy that night. Dennis turned off her television, and we turned on a nearby radio to a Christian station. I encouraged Joy to open her curtains in the morning and soak up the sunshine. We brought her water to drink and let her talk. After about an hour her crying stopped, and we prayed with her, claiming God's promise of peaceful sleep for Joy.

Why do I tell you this story? You and I were taught from childhood the importance of sleep—enough sleep. I enjoyed a mother and father who listened to my prayers at bedtime, read me a story, and tucked me in with a kiss. "Sleep helps you to grow," my mother often said, even as she must have thanked God for a few minutes of quietness from the demands of an active family.

In magazines and newspapers, over the radio, and in medical offices we are told that adults and children alike are *suffering* from a lack of sleep. "Sleep deprivation," they call it. This condition robs children of their ability to think clearly. Teens find their minds muddled when they miss their zzz's. You and I suffer too. Lack of sleep makes us grouchy. We become nervous or depressed. Sometimes we even walk into another room or get into the car and forget what we're there for. Could some of this forgetfulness also be sleep-related?

Do you resist sleep because of fear? Go to Psalm 3:5, 6: "I lay down and slept; I awoke, for the Lord sustained me. I will not be afraid of ten thousands of people who have set themselves against me all around."

Solomon shares another beautiful promise: "When you lie down, you will not be afraid; Yes, you will lie down and your sleep will be sweet" (Proverbs 3:24).

Solomon hurries on, though, and we understand his words better after viewing the horrors of death and destruction visited upon innocent people in Oklahoma City, New York City, Washington, D.C., and many other parts of the world. Repeat his words whenever distressful thoughts enter your mind: "Do not be afraid of sudden terror, nor of trouble from the wicked when it comes; for the Lord will be your confidence, and will keep your foot from being caught" (verses 25, 26).

Jesus Himself set the example as He slept soundly that dark and stormy night on the Sea of Galilee. He could. He created the sea, the night, the world. He controlled the storm (Mark 4:35-41; Matthew 14:22-33). But He also created you and me. And for our comfort and assurance He gave us the moon to light the night (Genesis 1:14-19).

What would you describe as the biggest robber of sleep—your sleep and mine? I think it's that we are. We find so much to see, so much to listen to, so much to do and experience. As a child does, I make excuses and trick myself into staying up later and later. *Just a few minutes more and I'll go to bed. One more segment of TV news. Fifteen more minutes of this exciting program. One more chore to finish. One more phone call to make or page to read in my magazine or book.* You have your own reasons and excuses to stay up. Each one—legitimate or imagined—has the ability to rob you of precious sleep.

At the other end of the spectrum are some of you that I picture shaking your head and wishing that not getting enough sleep were your problem. For you, the pain starts when you open your eyes. Sleeping at least brings relief from sorrow.

King David experienced so much in his lifetime. Listen to his words of comfort and hope: "O Lord my God, I cried out to You, and You healed me. O Lord, You brought my soul up from the grave; You have kept me alive, that I should not go down to the pit. Sing praise to the Lord, you saints of His, and give thanks at the remembrance of His holy name. For His anger is but for a moment, His favor is for life; Weeping may endure for a night, but joy comes in the morning" (Psalm 30:2-5).

There's more. "Oh, taste and see that the Lord is good; blessed is the man who trusts in Him" (Psalm 34:8). Perhaps it's time for you to taste God's goodness. Could it be time for you to turn from your sorrow and reach out to Another who also knows the loneliness of the path of sorrow and loss? Turn to Jesus. Trust in Him. "Joy comes in the morning"!

Reserve your energy.

It's that age-old story. Martha scurries around the kitchen with endless preparations to care for while Mary sits at Jesus' feet. I don't know which of them you relate to best, but I do know that I've been in both camps—serving and listening.

Children seem to come with a limitless supply of energy. In fact, Dennis and I often comment on how thankful we are that we raised our children when we were younger, because it takes all the energy we have to keep up with our grandchildren. Do you find yourself fading by the end of the day? Tiredness comes as we age. There will come a day when all of our senses grow dim and our life begins to fail.

Each new day comes with the opportunity to do just so much. You can squander your time and energy on things that matter little or you can plan your day wisely—everything from the steps you take (such as trips up the stairs and back down) to how often you indulge in times of fear and anger. You can enjoy each moment or you can despise your life. Your life may last 70 years or only 30. You may live a strong and healthy 100 years or a feeble and shaky 60 years.

"You do not know what will happen tomorrow. For what is your life? It is even a vapor that appears for a little time and then vanishes away. Instead you ought to say, 'If the Lord wills, we shall live and do this or that'" (James 4:14, 15). In everything, I keep foremost in my mind that God has a plan for my life. I find myself joining with Moses, saying, "Oh, satisfy us early with Your mercy, that we may rejoice and be glad all our days! Make us glad according to the days in which You have afflicted us, the years in which we have seen evil. Let Your work appear to Your servants, and Your glory to their children. And let the beauty of the Lord our God be upon us, . . . yes, establish the work of our hands" (Psalm 90:14-17).

In Ecclesiastes 3 we read that there's a time for everything. It's my time. It's your time. "But those who wait on the Lord shall renew their strength; they shall mount up with wings like eagles, they shall run and not be weary, they shall walk and not faint" (Isaiah 40:31). God and I will walk, run, and work together.

Resist **temptation.**

I knew that somewhere in the Bible God tells me to resist temptation. What a surprise I got when I found the passage. It goes like this: "Submit to God. Resist the devil and he will free from you. Draw near to God and He will draw near to you" (James 4:7, 8).

Submit to God? Submit before resisting? That sounds as if I can't resist temptation all alone. But then, if Eve couldn't, what makes me think I can do more than she?

"Resist" means to strive against, to act counter to, to withstand, to offer opposition.

To resist temptations we must acknowledge we are sinful and human. "I was brought forth in iniquity, and in sin my mother conceived me" (Psalm 51:5). We have to be able to recognize the devil and those associated with him. Most important, with God's help we must flee. Turn from temptation. Run the other way. Be careful not to let sin overtake us.

How hard is that? Hard enough, but our help is awesome! When we come near to God, let Him be our shepherd, He will lead us "in the paths of righteousness" (Psalm 23:3). "Goodness and mercy" will follow us all the days of our lives, and we "will dwell in the house of the Lord forever" (verse 6).

That's why I find that studying God, beholding God, and copying what God does are all ways to resist the devil. He walks about like a "roaring lion" (1 Peter 5:8), you know!

Refuel **with friendship and laughter.**

It's almost Thanksgiving. You and your family have decided to head out to spend the holiday with your parents or some special friends. Unfortunately, you leave home long after your planned departure time, and you feel tense as you slide behind the wheel. Heavy traffic, wind, and perhaps rain or snow all add to your discomfort. For a time you wonder about your good judgment. Could you really have believed this trip was a good idea? "I've been there and done that!" you say to me. Haven't we all? Late into the night you reach your destination, tired and thankful for a safe trip. After sharing a few quick greetings and warm hugs, the world of sleep overtakes you. *Tomorrow,* you think as you drift off, *tomorrow all this stress and weariness will be worth it.*

And tomorrow comes. A new day! Twenty-four hours to be lived with good food, rich laughter, and abundant joy. You are right. You'd do it again in the blink of an eye. What a blessing, this kicking back with those you love and care about brings you. It's no wonder that Jesus visited Peter's home and spent much time with Mary, Martha, and Lazarus.

From the garden forward, God knew His children. He wants each to enjoy the days He gives them, and to find "a time to laugh; . . . a time to embrace" (Ecclesiastes 3:4, 5).

---

*Not her real name.

Chapter Seven

GOD IN YOUR HEART

Trust in God's Guidance and Know His Healing Grace.

Job asked God the same questions you and I ask today. The hard questions we are often too afraid, distracted, or busy to ask: "What is man, that You should exalt him, that You should set Your heart on him, that You should visit him every morning, and test him every moment? How long? Will You not look away from me, and let me alone till I swallow my saliva?" (Job 7:17).

When it comes right down to it, what am I in this crowded world? Am I as a speck of dust? Does my very existence come to anything when all is said and done? What difference does it make how I live my life, one way or the other?

God did not answer Job right away, and I'm not surprised. It seems that God wanted him—He wants you and me—to figure out some things for ourselves. Perhaps He has in mind for me just to accept some things that I can't understand. Woven into my life are many such things. There certainly are questions: How can I know and understand God? Why would God care about me? Does God have a purpose for my life?

The list goes on and on. I grow tired and discouraged wondering . . . pondering . . . longing for purpose and meaning. That's were the next step comes in: trust in divine guidance.

Each of these laws of health interweaves with the others. When I focus completely on *any* one, I lose sight of the others—the whole picture. God wants me to become a whole creature. He sent *me* His Spirit. The presence of God must always be in my life or I will walk around with a gaping hole right where my heart should be.

If not for God's grace . . . what of me? "For by grace you have been saved through faith, and that not of yourselves; it is the gift of God, not of works, lest anyone should boast. For we are His workmanship, created in Christ Jesus for good works, which God prepared beforehand that we should walk in them" (Ephesians 2:8-10).

Read all of Ephesians 2. I marvel at the pictures Paul paints for me: "And you He made alive, who were dead in trespasses and sins, in which you once walked according to the course of this world, according to the prince of the power of the air, the spirit who now works in the sons of disobedience" (verses 1, 2).

It's almost more than I can take in. I want to know more. My life depends on it. I can't stop now. I need to know more about God's presence and guidance.

Take time for God and His Word.

I walked with a friend along a country road. We talked of God and our relationship with Him. She shared her habits of daily prayer and Bible study. My efforts seemed so meager and unacceptable.

Our conversation moved on to prayer. When did we each pray? How did we pray? With whom did we enjoy praying? She shared how God must grieve when we fail to talk to Him. I pondered that statement. How *does* God feel when I fail to make connection? Is He angry? Spiteful?

A couple days passed, and life settled into another hectic week. Still, in the far recesses of my mind hung the unanswered thoughts of God and prayer and our lack of it. One day while writing to a friend, I reached for the little book a friend gave me, *God Is in the Small Stuff,* by Bruce Bickel and Stan Jantz, and began to read slowly—here a page, there a page.

Suddenly my eyes fell on a short paragraph in the reading for September 18. My heart thrilled. I knew God was speaking directly to me through that page: "The good news is that God doesn't put conditions on your prayer life. His feelings don't get hurt when you don't pray. But when you do, He connects with you in a powerful way. Try it today. Try it right now. Talk to God. He's listening."

Pray without ceasing? Just as my husband, my children, are ever a part of the fiber of my being, so can God be. Yes, just as lessons, words, and examples my parents taught me come to mind at the most unexpected time, God will become an "in all things" part of my life.

Let me share a few pointers that I've found make my time with Him more special and more real. Add to these. Adapt them to your circumstances. Enjoy God. He surely does love us. We know this "because He laid down His life for us" (1 John 3:16).

Treasure **God's hand in your life.**

You and I come to this point of our lives having traveled different roads and encountered different circumstances. That's what makes your life—*you!* Your unique story. The material of that amazing song you will sing in heaven. No other man or woman lived just as you have lived.

Make it a part of your day to treasure God's hand in your life. Did you experience a rocky and unhappy childhood? Perhaps the depth of your compassion stems from this. Did you endure a painful marriage? How many others can benefit from the wisdom you learned in that valley?

Are you trying to forget the demons of destruction and

death? God says, "My grace is sufficient for you, for My strength is made perfect in weakness" (2 Corinthians 12:9). God's love never fails. He has promised to "never leave you nor forsake you" (Hebrews 13:5). He searches for you when you stray (Matthew 18:12). *You can trust Him with your life!*

Trust through tears of sorrow and times of joy.

Do not be surprised when bad things happen to you. Jesus says, "In the world you will have tribulation; but be of good cheer, I have overcome the world" (John 16:33). In Romans 12:12 we are instructed to be "patient in tribulation."

More than that, we are told in Romans 5:3, 4 to "glory in tribulations, knowing that tribulation produces perseverance; and perseverance, character; and character, hope." After Thessalonian Christians grew through their times of trial, Paul wrote to them, "We are bound to thank God always for you, brethren, as it is fitting, because your faith grows exceedingly, and the love of every one of you all abounds toward each other, so that we ourselves boast of you among the churches of God for your patience and faith in all your persecutions and tribulations that you endure, which is manifest evidence of the righteous judgment of God, that you may be counted worthy of the kingdom of God, for which you also suffer" (2 Thessalonians 1:3-5). He finishes by promising that God will "repay with tribulation those who trouble you" (verse 6).

From what I've learned of the human body and mind, we often forget the things that brought us so much grief and pain and remember the wonderful times. Let your mind wonder to the greatest times of your life. God's hand was there—even if you didn't see it. He loves to give us good and perfect gifts (James 1:17).

I celebrate God's love by growing flowers, cooking,

and sharing healthful food. I celebrate God's love by singing, walking, and at times crying for joy. How do you mark these times? "Watch what God does, and then you do it, like children who learn proper behavior from their parents. Mostly what God does is love you. Keep company with him and learn a life of love. Observe how Christ loved us. His love was not cautious but extravagant. He didn't love in order to get something from us but to give everything of Himself to us. Love like that" (Ephesians 5:1, 2, Message).

Tarry to look for tokens of God's love.

Should you read everything above this section and throw up your hands in despair, keep on reading and determine to begin here. Can you believe, after all these years of sin, the beauty of the world we live in? I live on the eastern side of the United States and love the seasons.

Spring! Ah, the colors that surprise and excite my senses every day. Frosty days turn slowly into balmy days. Wind blows, chimes ring, delightful smells fill the air. I can hardly bear to see spring turn into summer, this time is so perfect for me.

Yet summer has a glory all it's own. No more coats, gloves, and hats. Gardens to be planted! Grass to be mowed, fertilized, and mowed yet again. Trees leaf out and birds build nests and sing glorious songs of praise and gladness to their Father. Children, free from the constraints of school, laugh and play. Imagine yourself once again riding bikes with abandon, playing ball or tag or chase. Butterflies, bees, and hummingbirds show God's sense of humor and delight.

Long before I'm ready to give up the joys of summer, fall takes center stage. Fall is Dennis's favorite time of year. Leaves turn to glorious shades of red, orange, and yellow.

Squirrels bury their nuts with a passion. Flocks of birds pass over and land on ponds, just to take off again and resume their journey southward. Slowly days become shorter and the air cooler. Skies glow with color in the morning or stage outlandish sunsets in the evening. Leaves fly through the air planting exquisite colors wherever they land, covering grass and soil with a layer of protection. The earth prepares for winter, and stillness reigns.

Suddenly it's winter. Snowflakes fly deliciously around your head, landing on your nose and in your eyes. Wind whips sleet and endless snow on nearly abandoned streets, and almost-invisible trucks throw out salt to make the streets safe again. Children build snowmen and emit peals of laughter as they fall in the snow, only to jump up and exclaim in wonder over snow angels they have eagerly made.

From the North to the South, from the East to the West, God's love brings visions of wonder. Take in nature's massive mountains and lovely valleys. Wander about with your light in a dark cave. Enjoy a swim in the ocean. You have only begun. Consider the desert. Take in a city—people bustling here and there—hurrying to met a friend or fulfill a host of life's necessities.

The list goes on into infinity. Our homes, our children, our pets, our food, friends who make us laugh. Cars, planes, and trains that enable us to travel to far away places. Sleep when we're weary. Energy when we awaken. Water, sun, shade, grass, and trees . . .

All these tokens of God's love are called blessings. As the song says: "Count your blessings, name them one by one, count your many blessings, see what God has done." "Hard" describes being anywhere and not being able to pick out a blessing. Open our eyes, Lord, to see them!

***Test* your beliefs and teach them to your children.**

The testing process begins on the day we are born. "Suck, baby, so you can be fed." So we practice and practice. "Why are you crying, baby? Let's see if we can figure out your needs." And we are comforted. "Can you crawl and walk, baby?" So we take a wobbly step and then another—testing ourselves and building strength again and again.

Now, as growing children, young adults, thirtysome-things, middle-aged men and women, or seniors, we continue to grow and test ourselves. We're never "good enough." We want to grow.

So also we must test our beliefs in God. "Why does God allow suffering?" someone asks. "Is God real?" another wants to know. "Should I pay tithes and give offerings?" your children ask themselves until they finally settle the issue for themselves.

"Are we on the path toward heaven?"

"What more can we do?"

"On what day of the week will we worship?"

"How can I find hope and assurance when I'm grieving the loss of my friend/loved one?"

"Why can't I be the one to get even, God? You know how hard these malicious rumors about my family and me have been on us."

"What about my job?"

"Why this sickness and pain?"

God must have understood our dilemmas when He gave us the Bible and encouraged us to study the Scriptures (2 Timothy 2:15), promising that "all Scripture is given by inspiration of God, . . . and is profitable" (2 Timothy 3:16).

Even as I answer these questions and many others for myself, I must teach these truths to my children. The devil will take every measure available to him to drag our children into sin and despair. Our only hope can be found in filling their minds with the love of Jesus. This hope will give a purpose for living to our sons and daughters, our grandchildren, godchildren, or those precious, seeking children attending a Vacation Bible School program for the first time. Our words of wisdom and encouragement may help keep them safe in a world of sin.

Team up with others.

Do you ever feel helpless or frightened? Imagine God calling to Moses before the burning bush, "Moses, Moses!"

And Moses answers, "Here I am."

The conversation becomes serious quickly. God wants to send Moses on a mission. Moses declines for many reasons. Finally, in desperation, Moses gets to the big excuse, "O my Lord, I am not eloquent, neither before nor since You have spoken to Your servant; but I am slow of speech and slow of tongue" (Exodus 4:10). Sound familiar? I know I've used that excuse enough times.

God does not seem to even hesitate, but responds, "Who has made man's mouth? Or who makes the mute, the deaf, the seeing, or the blind? Have not I, the Lord? Now therefore, go, and I will be with your mouth and teach you what you shall say" (verses 11, 12). Moses still wasn't buying it.

"O my Lord," he pleads, "please send by the hand of whomever else You may send" (verse 13).

God's angry reply comes in an instant, "Is not Aaron the Levite your brother? I know that he can speak well. And look, he is also coming out to meet you. When he sees you, he will be glad in his heart. Now you shall speak to him and put the words in his mouth. And I will be with your mouth and with his mouth, and I will teach you what you shall do. So he shall be your spokesman to the people. And he himself shall be as a mouth for you, and you shall be to him as God" (verses 14-16).

Throughout the Bible we see teamwork again and again. Prayer partners move mountains. Leaders and teachers help each other spread the story of Christ. Young and old work together when neither has the courage to go it alone. The educated and self-taught reach out as one to make the world a better place. Two are stronger than one; a threefold cord cannot easily be broken, the Wise Man says.

Tread softly, for temptations abound.

When we're little they call it "showing off." We hold our head up high and endeavor to perform impossible feats of skill and daring. In the end we fall on our face, or some other calamity befalls us.

I've found as an adult that I often grab my hand away from God's, and as my nose rises skyward I let Him know in no uncertain terms, "I can do it myself. Just leave me alone. I don't need you telling me what to do!"

Imagine the joy of the devil. "This one's on her own. Hit it! She's easy prey." Defenses down, I fall into various temptations that bring me much grief and suffering. If only I'd had my hand in His. If only . . .

Peter found out the hard way. "Well, Lord, I'll never betray you. You can count on me." "Let me walk to You, Lord. Look, I'm doing it!" Abraham found out the hard way. "My wife? You've got to be kidding. This beautiful woman is my sister!" David found out the hard way. "She's beautiful. I want her."

Adam and Eve suffered when they decided to go it alone. Jonah's running-away experience left much to be desired. Samson could have avoided so much pain and suffering if only he had followed the way God outlined for him.

What about you? How closely are you walking with God? How many times are you going to fall because you looked away from the one who guides your footsteps?

You choose. Even when you've looked away and find yourself battered and bruised, stand up and let God direct your steps. You can trust Him.

Taste of God's goodness.

When was the last time you did something nice for someone you cared about? Did you enjoy it? Did they appreciate it? Will it be your last time?

Silly questions? Yet I find myself thinking of God as a stern sergeant waiting to catch me off guard and punish me in the cruelest of way. Unreasonable? Yes, I know that. Yet there have been times when I have been stern and unbending. It's very easy to think of God as being like me.

My boss calls me in and gives me a well-deserved raise, and I can hardly hold back my joy and appreciation. A friend shares some of her bounty from her overflowing garden, and I'm so thankful that I can't say enough good things about it. The doctor gives me a clean bill of health, and I tell everyone I know.

But God creates a beautiful world, fills it with every good thing imaginable, and I sit quietly by, hardly reaching out my hand to enjoy all these bounties.

I find myself appreciating God the most when I've prayed for someone who is sick, and the fever breaks and they sleep quietly, whereas moments before they struggled for breath. When I've encouraged a stranger or visited those who are lonely or in prison, God has seemed very near. As an "encourager" I know God's joy in serving. As the recipient of another of God's daughters' love and encouragement, I feel His touch and am comforted.

Chapter Eight

THE CONCLUSION OF THE MATTER

The Secret of Success—Abstinence and Moderation

As a child growing up in Loma Linda, California, my husband, Dennis, enjoyed trips. Mile after mile passed by, and he watched and learned. The trip home took so long, though. Would the car make it that far? Would they run out of gas? These questions and more filled the mind of the little boy. Suddenly, as the groaning car rounded the last turn, his little voice could always be heard from the back seat of the car: "Look, Dad. It's OK now. We can walk home from here!"

Each day that we are granted makes up part of our journey. What you put into every 24-hour period will forever be a part of your history. This day—the one you're eager to enjoy, hoping to avoid, or living with abandon—will take its place in your life's story, for better or worse.

You can choose the components that make up each one. Today you can be a blessing or you can use your voice (or your horn) to curse another. You can spend your time working hard and going the second mile or you can spend it in gossip and indecision. You see, you hold the reigns—unless you hand them over to God. That decision, to let God sit in the driver's seat, can be scary, though. "'For My thoughts are not your thoughts, nor are your ways My ways,' says the Lord" (Isaiah 55:8).

You must decide. If you are a child, you will have to obey the adults whose hands your life is placed in. But as an adult, you're the one with the choice. That brings us to the last of the laws of physical and spiritual health—abstinence and moderation—and gives us more choices to make.

Abstinence and moderation don't seem so hard, do they? It's not hard for me to think *This may be my easiest challenge yet. You see, I have many good qualities. I usually talk softly and smile a lot. I try to eat right and get my exercise whenever possible. What else could be expected of me?*

If so, I'm kidding myself. I'm a weak woman. I must be related to the apostle Paul. Surely "the good that I will to do, I do not do; but the evil I will not to do, that I practice" (Romans 7:19). If Paul, after all those years of service for Christ, still could say things like that, what hope do I have? But wasn't it also Paul who went on to use that "do" word in another way when he said, "I can *do* all things through Christ who strengthens me" (Philippians 4:13)?

Let's see where our journey with Christ takes us last.

Avoid excess, even in that which is good.

That's a pretty clear picture. It sort of reminds me of what Paul says in 1 Corinthians 10:31, which includes that little word "do" again: "Whether you eat or drink, or whatever you do, *do* all to the glory of God."

I've got it. It's really important for me to pay attention to everything I do. My life should not be like a roller-coaster with a succession of too much and then too little. It should be balanced.

No matter what I'm doing, wearing, eating, drinking, watching, or hearing, I can't go on doing it forever without stealing time, energy, and/or resources from some other part of my life. If I skip walking, my body will become weak. If I walk after I feel the pain of blisters forming, I will pay in pain and suffering.

Should I decide to take my work to the excess—to put in long days and weekends—I will pay by losing the enjoyment and friendship of my family and friends. Eat until I am sick and tired, and I will reap sickness and suffering. H'mmm! It's not a pretty picture. I think I get the point!

Accept that you will reap the effects of over indulgence or disobedience.

Sounds a lot like avoiding excess to me. The Bible seems very clear on this one, and I can imagine that Paul speaks from experience when he says that "whatever a man sows, that will he also reap" (Galatians 6:7).

The story is told of two children who loved to visit their grandparents and stay with them for a few weeks each summer. Dan especially enjoyed sitting on the tractor, riding the horses, and helping to milk the cows. Jody couldn't get enough of petting the cats, chasing the kittens, and gathering eggs. They both liked the swinging in the front-porch swing.

Their visits would have been perfect, except for one thing.

Their Gram insisted that both of them be ready for bed, tucked in (even though it seemed too hot for covers), and their prayers said by 8:00. Every night! Without fail! It wasn't fair. They weren't even tired. In fact, it wasn't even dark outside yet.

It didn't matter. No matter how many times they begged and pleaded with her, Gram wouldn't budge.

One night, just before darkness settled in and quite a while before Gram made her nightly check, Dan got an idea.

"Jody, are you asleep yet?" he whispered loudly.

"Not yet!" she whispered back. "I'm not even tired."

"I've got an idea." *Silence*.

Dan crossed quietly into Jody's bedroom. "Let's crawl out on the roof and eat an apple. I can reach some easily from there. Let's try one. Come on!"

"I don't know." Jody hesitated. "Gram won't like it. She'll be very unhappy and punish us for sure if she finds out. You know how she always says that eating between meals will make us sick and ruin our appetites."

"No way! Besides, she won't ever know." Dan could almost taste the juicy apple. "Come on, Jody. Don't be such a fraidy-cat!"

Quietly they opened the window and crawled out onto the roof. Dan crawled carefully over to the edge and reached for a *big* apple. He wiped it on his pajama leg and handed it to Jody.

"It does taste good." she giggled. "I was getting hungry. You'd better try one too."

Already Dan had a second apple in his grasp, polishing it with great anticipation. The first ones tasted so good that they both had another.

Just in time they crawled into their beds and pretended to be asleep when the door opened slightly for Gram's last "good night" to the sleeping children.

Early the next morning Dan sat up and stretched. Did he feel sick? Had the apples ruined his appetite? He felt no ill effects. Quickly he crossed the hall and peeked into Jody's room.

"Wake up!" he called to Jody. "Are you all right? Does your stomach hurt?"

"No!" She yawned and giggled.

Satisfied that neither had suffered any ill effects, they both dressed quickly and went happily down to breakfast. Gram's pancakes had never tasted better. The strawberries they ate tasted sweet as sugar.

Soon the events of the night before were forgotten.

That evening after the dishes were done, Dan and Jody, eager to put off their bedtime, climbed into the porch swing. Suddenly Dan jumped off and ran to the other side of the porch.

"Let's have another apple before bedtime," he teased.

"I don't know—we could get caught," Jody stammered.

Already Dan was reaching high into the nearest branch for an extra-big apple. He gave it a quick swipe across his leg and took a bite. *Wonderful,* he thought. *This is great!*

Just before taking a second bite he looked down at the apple. Suddenly his stomach leaped into his throat. It couldn't be. It wasn't possible! Yet there, as plain as the shoes on his feet lay, not a worm, but half a worm.

He spit. He sputtered. He felt sick. Nothing could take away the awful feeling. A closer check showed both children the dreaded and awful truth—the apples were all full of worms.

Perhaps you've lived your life in the same way that I've lived mine. You try to make the right choices, but sometimes you just can't seem to help yourself, and you give in to choices that you know could be harmful. What a feeling of relief you get when the hours, days, and even years pass and it seems you've "gotten away with it"!

Jesus says that we will reap what we sow. Perhaps it won't even be in our lifetime, but in the lives of our children or others who follow our example. Each choice we make has a consequence. Determine to make your choices wisely—with God.

Account for the life you live.

Have you ever wanted to hide? Perhaps an experiment you tried turned out all wrong. Who of us hasn't gotten into a jam and looked around to see if anyone has seen us. *Perhaps I can just sneak away and no one will know I did it,* we say to ourselves.

There are times we can even say that we *did* get away with it. No, it's not something any of us can be proud of, but at the time it surely did beat facing the music. The only trouble is, scars of deceit can't be washed away that easily. Even when others don't find out, we know—and God knows.

I often laugh at our cats. Our 20-pound Bear cat is the worst. He'll jump onto a table in front of the window and in doing so knock down a book. Instead of looking guilty, he just sits looking happily out the window as if nothing had ever happened.

On this earth we can try to turn away from, ignore, or lie about the sins we have committed. But in heaven the story is different. "'As I live, says the Lord, every knee shall bow to Me, and every tongue shall confess to God.' So then each of us shall give account of himself to God" (Romans 14:11, 12).

Anchor **your life.**

In our backyard stands a maple tree. You wouldn't exactly call it beautiful. It's not very full, but the squirrels do seem to enjoy it. We lament that unlike many other trees in our yard, it doesn't seem to turn pretty colors in the fall.

"Then why do you keep it?" you ask. "Why not take it out?"

A tree cutter checked all of the trees in our yard a few years ago to make sure they wouldn't blow over in the wind and damage our house. He focused in on the backyard maple.

"This tree needs to be anchored," he announced. "It's a great shade tree and probably does a lot to keep this side of your house cool."

What a difference that strong cable made. The two branches that had separated close to the bottom no longer faced the danger of splitting apart. We've often gazed at that particular tree and felt that fortifying it turned out to be money well spent.

What keeps your life from splitting apart? A better question would be Who keeps you safe and satisfied? Do you find yourself changing directions whenever the winds of strife blow? Could tribulation batter and scar your exterior, causing irreversible damage?

Just as Dennis and I experienced firsthand the importance of maintaining the tree that we love, it's even more important to do everything possible to anchor ourselves and those we love.

The anchor can be found in Hebrews 6:19: "This hope we have as an anchor of the soul, both sure and steadfast." In Him I find calm amid the storm. Clinging to Jesus, I can even become a refuge for others who are seeking and searching, often ready to let go when their strength is gone.

Jesus is our Rock. He is our Refuge. As a mother hen He longs to gather us under His wings when danger approaches. We can count on Him as our shelter in the time of storm. We cannot hide from Him. He's powerful, to be praised, and full of compassion. He's altogether lovely.

Begin your search today. Assemble a picture of the Man of Galilee. He's calling to you, "Come to Me, all you who labor and are heavy laden," so He can give you rest (Matthew 11:28). Need comfort? He's there for you. Are you afraid of failing? Seek His face. Seeking love? "God is love" (1 John 4:8).

Ask yourself if "almost" really is good enough.

How often have you quoted the well-known sentence "A miss is as good as a mile"?

That may be true when it comes to avoiding an accident, a ticket, or that pothole, deer, or piece of tire in the road. These misses make the most exciting stories. "There we were, just coming around the curve, when he stepped out in front of us. . . . My daughter closed her eyes; and I slammed on the brakes. . . . That was some large beast. . . . He could have done in both of us."

It isn't that way in the spiritual realm, for those of us who have our eyes focused on heaven. The five foolish virgins "almost" had enough oil. The guest at the wedding feast could have been wearing a robe "almost" like the one the host had given him to wear, but he didn't, and without the correct robe he was thrown into utter darkness. Peter "almost" walked successfully on the water. Moses "almost" followed God's instruction when he struck the rock. So many stories, so many "almost, but not quite" events. Yet in each case something went amiss.

Almost is not good enough. "Almost" means we've tried to make it on our own without the most important ingredient—Jesus, the Son of God. "Almost" describes the goats rather than the sheep, the tares rather than the wheat, the rich young ruler rather than the disciples. It's not good enough. "Then Agrippa said to Paul, 'You almost persuade me to become a Christian'" (Acts 26:28). Such sad words!

"Almost" must turn into "all." "All to Jesus I surrender, all to Him I freely give." "Though He slay me, yet will I trust Him" (Job 13:15). Even as Stephen lay down his life willingly for the Lord, praying for those who stoned him, so we must trust Him with everything. Nothing can be held apart from Him. When we relinquish our lives into His keeping, we can say with the apostle Paul, "We both labor and suffer reproach, because we trust in the living God, who is the Savior of all men, especially of those who believe" (1 Timothy 4:10).

Acknowledge that abundance can be a curse and a killer.

You've done it. I've done it too. Each day we scrimp,

save, wish, and hope. Often we overspend or borrow for an abundance of "treasures." Yet the Bible tells us, "Do not lay up for yourselves treasures on earth, where moth and rust destroy and where thieves break in and steal; but lay up for yourselves treasures in heaven, where neither moth nor rust destroys and where thieves do not break in and steal. For where your treasure is, there your heart will be also" (Matthew 6:19-21).

An abundance of possessions often force us to invest in still more things. They draw us into a vicious cycle. Yet which of them bring joy and peace into my life? Can I look at my overabundance and say "These things draw me closer to the Lord"? When I find myself spending more and more time seeking things instead of God, I must stop immediately and refocus.

What can be more important than my connection with God? Why would I want to continue to buy more, worry more, work harder for things that only separate me from a life hid in Christ? Ask yourself this question: Do I own anything that will separate me from God? Which of my belongings am I not willing to give up, if the Spirit impresses me, for the sake of eternal life?

If you answer truly that everything you own has been dedicated to God, you are walking, perhaps running, toward God.

Does your house belong to Him? Whom do you honor with your office and car? I don't mean they must be small and stripped of all earthly comforts. Surely Job didn't drive the cheapest vehicle—after all, he had a large family. But do our possessions bless others? Or do they grow dusty and rusty while we labor for more and still more?

Can my life lived apart from the Creator, simply because I've become too wrapped up in temporal things to spend quality time with Him, be real and lasting? Will I find eternal life in a large-screen television? What can I gain or give to others from my fast car or luxurious boat? Do they lead me into the world and its ways, or draw me closer to Christ?

Humility cures worldliness. James 4:8 tells us, "Draw near to God and He will draw near to you." Which of your possessions cause you to ignore God? Study the real root of temptation. "Let no one say when he is tempted, 'I am tempted by God'; for God cannot be tempted by evil, nor does He himself tempt anyone. But each one is tempted when he is drawn away by his own desires and enticed" (James 1:13, 14).

Sounds a bit like Eve—and Adam. Brings to mind the rich young ruler and the Pharisees. "So when Jesus heard these things, He said to him [the rich young ruler], 'You still lack one thing. Sell all that you have and distribute to the poor, and you will have treasure in heaven; and come, follow Me.' But when he heard this, he became very sorrowful, for he was very rich" (Luke 18:22, 23).

Possessions can place us in the position of wanting more and better for the sake of having and impressing. Pursuit of them can create pride and thievery. Abraham had many things but became a nomad for God. Job had much, but lost all. Peter, John, and the other disciples were willing to give up everything when the call came to follow Jesus.

Maintain a readiness—even an eagerness—to obey God's will in your life. Foster a willingness—a burning desire—to serve Him. Develop a steadfastness to follow His will. Pledge to God that you will follow Him whenever and wherever He leads. These are the attributes God desires.

No one can be the conscience for another. I cannot judge the rightness or wrongness of your personal belongings or how you relate to them. Each of us must answer only for ourselves. Your shortcomings are known only to you and to God. You alone can invite God to direct your life completely.

"Turn your eyes upon Jesus, look full in His wonderful face; and the things of earth will grow strangely dim in the light of His glory and grace." The words of the beloved hymn still ring true today.

The way you live, the choices you make—look to Christ for direction in these areas. God's "word is a lamp to [your] feet and a light to [your] path" (Psalm 119:105). Your walk will be unique. Throughout your life, your days will include hills and valleys. You will walk through deserts and ford streams. Some days may find you feeling lost and experiencing deep loneliness. Ah, but there will be others that include "walking on water" and flying to new heights.

Avoid **addiction.**

You've heard the words. Perhaps you've even said some of them: "A day's just not a day without . . ." "Let's hurry home, it's almost time for . . ." "We never miss watching [attending, listening to] . . ." These are just a few of the statements that give us a hint that we've become addicted. Something other than Christ drives our life.

It's easy to think of drinking, smoking, gambling, and drugs as addictions. Yet these are just a few of the areas in which we fall into destructive lifestyles. Any area of our life may lead us into addiction. It may well be the desire to control others. Or to clean the house all hours of the day and night. Or to buy and cook more food than our family can possibly eat.

I've met men and women who are addicted to their work, to excessive vacations, or to certain kinds of music. There's more. Our lips and tongues often become obsessed with talking about others—telling tales filled with untruths or misleading statements. Some folks find sleeping around the clock on holidays and weekends a misguided relief from responsibility or perhaps even pain. It's easier to hide from our demons rather than face them.

Anything, taken to excess, becomes a harmful activity. Too much food, television, or fun and games harms, rather than builds up, our bodies. An overabundance of education without work, relaxation, and sustenance can only wreak havoc on our systems.

Our guidebook must be only the Bible. I love to read Psalm 37. My version calls this chapter "The Heritage of the Righteous and the Calamity of the Wicked."

Keep your mind clear. Philippians 4:5 says, "Let your moderation be known unto all men. The Lord is at hand" (KJV). "Whatever things are true, . . . whatever things are just, whatever things are pure, whatever things are lovely, whatever things are of good report, if there is any virtue and if there is anything praiseworthy—meditate on these things" (verse 8).

Achieve in all areas to win the race.

The song says, "The things of earth will grow strangely dim." What brings on that dimness? Are we seeking for dim vision?

As I walk toward the light of God, the things of earth will lose their luster. No longer do I find my pattern for living by following the example of fellow travelers—I look to Jesus. He anoints my eyes with salve so I can see (Revelation 3:18). My experience on the Damascus road turns me toward God, and I long to go forward sharing the truth of God's love with others, without fear.

I may see Jesus in the fire, as did Moses. Perhaps He will speak to me in visions or dreams, as He did to the boy Samuel, Joseph, Peter, and John. I will follow, trusting His will to become plain as I go steadfastly along my journey. "The Lord will scatter you among the peoples, and you will be left few in number among the nations where the Lord will drive you" (Deuteronomy 4:27). "You will seek the Lord your God, and you will find Him if you seek Him with all your heart and with all your soul" (verse 29).

God loves you and me enough to die for us (John 3:16). Now we must love Him enough to live for Him. Whatever we do—eat, drink; it doesn't matter—it must *all* be done to the glory of God (1 Corinthians 10:31).

Someday we will understand. Everything! "God will wipe away every tear from their eyes; there shall be no more death, nor sorrow, nor crying. There shall be no more pain, for the former things have passed away" (Revelation 21:4). We're not in this earthly battle alone. We do not wrestle against flesh and blood (Ephesians 6:12). "He who endures to the end will be saved" (Matthew 10:22).

"Grow in the grace and knowledge of our Lord and Savior Jesus Christ. To Him be the glory both now and forever. Amen" (2 Peter 3:18).

Appendix A

MAKE YOUR TIME WITH GOD MORE SPECIAL

What do you want from your time with God? Think about your devotional life. What's the best part? If you could make it better, what would you do? We do not glorify God or fall in love with Him when we study "because we have to" or "the way we always did." As we live, each moment alters our understanding. The way we see and interpret things that happen around us changes moment by moment. We see life through a different grid because we constantly have new experiences. See God out of new eyes and make your learning fresh. Pretend you have the eyes of a child. Give the Holy Spirit opportunity to "open your mind."

1. Start reading a new version of the Bible. (Open your mind to new ideas.)
2. Envision a living God. (Risen and rejoicing in your love.)
3. Check your trust level. (Full or barely there?)
4. Question how you view God. (Make a list of your favorite texts describing God.)
5. Study God's view of you. (List all texts you find describing how God feels about you.)
6. Learn to listen to God. (How does He talk to you?)
7. Give God more of your time. (Throughout the day, pray and commune with Him.)
8. Keep a book of promises.
9. Keep a book of answered prayers.
10. Keep a book of miracles in your life, your friends' lives, and your family members' lives.

11. Share what you know about God with others. (When we get full enough of God's love, it spills over and out of us.)

12. Become a prayer warrior. Find a friend and unite your prayers in God's name. In the garden, Jesus longed for His friends to join Him in His prayer for strength.

13. Take better care of yourself. (A glowing life focuses away from us and on God.)

14. Let go of fear. (All of it.)

15. Learn to love like God does. (The sinner—not the sin. Judge not, lest you be judged.)

16. Copy what God does for you as you live your life.

"THE LITTLE TEACUP"

⌒

There was a couple who loved to go to England and shop in the little specialty stores. They both liked antiques and china, and especially teacups. One day they came across a delightful little shop in which they saw a beautiful teacup. They said to the salesclerk, "May we see that? We've never seen one quite so beautiful."

As the woman handed it to them, suddenly the teacup spoke. "You don't understand," it said, "I haven't always been a teacup. There was a time when I was red and I was clay. My Master took me and rolled me and patted me all over, and I yelled, "Stop it! Leave me alone!" But He only smiled and said, "Not yet."

Then I was placed on a spinning wheel, and suddenly I was spun around and around and around. "Quit it this instant," I screamed. "I'm getting dizzy!" But the Master only nodded and said, "Not yet." Then He put me in the oven. I never felt such heat. I wondered why he wanted to burn me. I yelled and yelled and pounded on the door. I could see Him through the opening, and I could read His lips as He shook His head and said, "Not yet."

Finally the door opened, He put me on the shelf, and I began to cool. "There, that's a whole lot better," I said. But then He took me down and began to brush and paint me all over. The fumes were horrible. I thought I would gag. "Stop it! Stop it!" I cried. He only nodded and said, "Not yet."

Then suddenly He put me back into the oven, not like the first one . . . oh, no! This one was twice as hot, and I just knew I would suffocate. I begged . . . I pleaded . . . I screamed . . . I cried . . . *I got angry!* All the time I could see Him through the opening, just nodding His head and saying, "Not yet."

Then I knew there wasn't any hope. I would never make it. I couldn't possibly endure this kind of punishment. I was ready to give up, but the door opened, and He took me out and placed me on the shelf again.

An hour later He handed me a mirror and said, "Look at yourself." And I did. I said, "That's not me! That couldn't be me! It's beautiful . . . I'm beautiful!"

"I want you to remember this," He said. "I know it hurts to be rolled and patted, but if I had left you alone, you'd have dried up. I know it made you dizzy to spin around and around on the wheel, but if I had stopped, you would have crumpled.

"I know it hurt and was hot and disagreeable in the oven, but if I hadn't put you there, you would have cracked. I know the fumes were bad when I brushed and painted you, but if I hadn't done that, you never would have hardened. You wouldn't have had any color in your life.

"And if I hadn't put you back in that second oven, you wouldn't have survived for very long, because the hardness wouldn't have held. Now you are a finished product. You are exactly what I had in mind when I first began with you."

When life seems to be spinning you around and around and you've been in the oven one too many times, think about the story of the little teacup. Remember that your life is in the hands of the Master Potter, who is not only making a beautiful creation out of you, but is also preparing you for life on this earth, and most of all for heaven.

—Author Unknown

Dear Reader,

In your daily walk toward wholeness and completeness, you may want to remember promises, lessons, and other encouraging bits of information you encounter. Jot them down on the following pages.

FRESH AIR

God's surprises to me come in these packages . . .

_____

_____

_____

_____

_____

_____

_____

_____

_____

_____

_____

_____

_____

SUNSHINE

I am blessed with . . . and I passed the blessings on to . . .

_____

_____

_____

_____

_____

_____

_____

_____

_____

_____

_____

_____

_____

_____

_____

GOOD FOOD

My "recipe" ideas and helpful hints for a more vibrant life . . .

_____

_____

_____

_____

_____

_____

_____

_____

_____

_____

_____

_____

_____

_____

_____

_____

_____

_____

EXERCISE

I've learned from my walk with God . . .

_____

_____

_____

_____

_____

_____

_____

_____

_____

_____

_____

_____

_____

_____

_____

_____

WATER

What I can't do without in my spiritual life . . . I sought the Lord, and He inclined His ear to me by . . .

_____

_____

_____

_____

_____

_____

_____

_____

_____

_____

_____

_____

_____

_____

_____

REST

I've taken the time to . . .

_____

_____

_____

_____

_____

_____

_____

_____

_____

_____

_____

_____

_____

_____

_____

_____

_____

TRUST IN DIVINE GUIDANCE

Father, I adore Thee because . . .

_____

_____

_____

_____

_____

_____

_____

_____

_____

_____

_____

_____

_____

_____

_____

_____

_____

ABSTINENCE AND MODERATION

When I fail and am discouraged, I . . .

_____

_____

_____

_____

_____

_____

_____

_____

_____

_____

_____

_____

_____

_____

_____

_____